'While it is often said that we learn more from our mistakes than our successes, few analysts dare to revisit what went wrong. Beth Feldman, however, boldly steps into that space, offering nine riveting case studies from her clinical practice. With rare transparency, she invites readers behind the closed doors of the therapy room and into the mind of an analyst grappling with the emotional and intellectual challenges of treatment – both during and long after it ends. Feldman's gift for storytelling shines on every page, guiding us through moments of laughter, tears, anxiety, and awe as we witness the profound transformations that reshape both therapist and patient.'

Danielle Knafo, Ph.D., *psychoanalyst, professor, author*

Case Studies in Relational Psychotherapy and Psychoanalysis

This book brings the reader behind the closed door of the psychotherapy office through a selection of nine riveting psychotherapy and psychoanalytic case studies.

Each story delves into the hearts and minds of memorable patients and their therapist as they grapple with loss, betrayal, anxiety, depression, suicidality, substance abuse, and more. With a strong relational focus, the author examines the misattunements, ruptures, and enactments that occurred in each treatment and explores in each case what she might have done differently – if she could turn back time. Each story is brought to life with her warm, empathic style and honest reflections as she shares her thoughts, feelings, reveries, and clinical decision-making in the treatment room. The myriad emotional challenges in each case study will resonate deeply with anyone who has been in therapy and with both new and seasoned clinicians.

With a warm and accessible style and wonderful attention to detail, this book is essential reading for psychoanalysts and psychotherapists wanting to get a better understanding of how to work with challenging patients and for anyone interested in understanding the unique challenges of psychoanalytic work.

Beth I. Feldman, Ph.D., is a clinical psychologist and relational psychoanalyst with a private practice in Plainview, New York. She treats adults and adolescents in individual, couples, and group therapy. Beth is the co-host of the podcast "Being a Parent Is Hard!" She is adjunct faculty at Post Graduate Program in Psychotherapy and Psychoanalysis, Derner Institute, Adelphi University. Beth has two adult children and lives with her husband and three dogs.

Case Studies in Relational Psychotherapy and Psychoanalysis

If I Could Turn Back Time

Beth I. Feldman

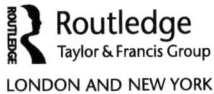
Routledge
Taylor & Francis Group

LONDON AND NEW YORK

First published 2025
by Routledge
4 Park Square, Milton Park, Abingdon, Oxon OX14 4RN

and by Routledge
605 Third Avenue, New York, NY 10158

Routledge is an imprint of the Taylor & Francis Group, an informa business

© 2025 Beth I. Feldman

British Library Cataloguing-in-Publication Data
A catalogue record for this book is available from the British Library

ISBN: 978-1-032-89542-0 (hbk)
ISBN: 978-1-032-89251-1 (pbk)
ISBN: 978-1-003-54334-3 (ebk)

DOI: 10.4324/9781003543343

Typeset in Optima
by Apex CoVantage, LLC

Jack, this book could only be dedicated to you. Over the years, you have been endlessly and selflessly supportive of my every interest and ambition – dogs, graduate school, dogs, analytic training, dogs, traveling, and most recently, my podcast and especially, my writing. Thank you for understanding me, indulging me, and believing in me, every step of the way.

Contents

Acknowledgements

I would like to thank my writing mentor, Dr. Danielle Knafo, for her unwavering support and her tireless guidance on every page of this book. She was relentlessly encouraging and helped me through my ambivalence about writing theory and my struggles with grammar and punctuation. I'd like to thank the members of our writing group, Joan Lipton, Ph.D., Melinda Blitzer, Ph.D., Alan Weiss, Ph.D., and Sheila Levi, Ph.D., for their ongoing support and encouragement. Joan, I am grateful for your ability to understand what I was trying to say, even when I wasn't clearly saying it, and for your unfailing warmth and positivity. Thank you, Melinda, for being the repetition police and catching any lack of clarity in my writing. Alan, I appreciate your calling out what didn't make sense and offering perfect, alternate ways of phrasing my ideas. And Sheila, thank you for challenging me theoretically and suggesting different ways of understanding the clinical work. I would like to express my gratitude to my first editor, Keith Talbot, for his encouragement, his guidance in sculpting the different versions of this book, and for helping me become a true writer. Many, many thanks to Catherine for always asking, always listening, and always offering her support and encouragement. Finally, I am so grateful to all my patients for inviting me into their lives, for trusting me, and for offering me the privilege of working with them.

Notice of Privacy

All the personal and identifying data of the patients described in the book have been significantly altered to maintain their confidentiality and anonymity. In several instances, the cases described are a composite of several patients. Similarly, the dialogue described has also been altered.

Introduction

Introduction

Six weeks into my internship at a prestigious psychiatric hospital, I had a moment as a young trainee that would influence me for years to come. It was a brisk fall day, and I was sitting on a bench with one of my most intimidating supervisors, trying desperately to appear more confident than I was feeling. Dr. Flynn was several decades older than I was, and he had an instinct for sniffing out anxiety in patients and trainees alike. I felt a surge of panic when he locked eyes with me and asked in his stern, deep voice, "Are you doing this work because you want to mother people or control them?"

"I want to help people," my thoughts pleaded, but I stayed silent, knowing this was not the answer he was looking for.

Once my "deer in the headlights" reaction subsided, he firmly instructed me: "The only correct answer is 'both.'"

This was a watershed moment, so early in my clinical career, in which I learned that it's okay to have strong feelings about my patients and conflicting motivations for much of what I say and do as a therapist. Most importantly, I learned that being aware of these strong feelings and how my inner world may spill into the treatment room makes me a better therapist.

Through decades of clinical work and analytic training, I have come to realize just how complicated the answer to my supervisor's question really is. I have come to understand that my strong feelings about my patients are the central, binding threads in the fabric of our relationship. These feelings are often a silent force, driving the emotional dramas that emerge between us. And they are vital to the curative power of our connection.

Over the years, there have been times I have wanted to hug my patients and moments I have wanted to hurt them, at times in the very way they had been hurt throughout their lives. Harsh words have occasionally escaped my mouth, and subtle grimaces have belied what I was feeling in the moment. I realized, however, that my patients did not need me to be perfect or unemotional. Quite the contrary. Today, I believe that they need me to care deeply enough to dive headfirst into their world, even if it means risking making mistakes. They need me to work hard to understand the complexity

DOI: 10.4324/9781003543343-1

of who they truly are and how they have come to be this way. And they need to feel that I too have some skin in the game – that I am willing to sweat and stumble along with them in their search for understanding and their fight for change.

My Book

This book offers more than a peek behind the closed door of my psycho-therapy office. I'll be shining a bright light into the memorable treatments of eight individual patients and one couple while also examining my own thoughts, feelings, reveries, and clinical decision-making in the treatment room. Join me as I try to feel, think, and experience the world as I imagine each patient does. In each case, I'll be focusing on the misattunements, rup-tures, and enactments that both thwarted our work and propelled the treat-ment forward. I'll muse about the paths taken as well as those not taken in each treatment. And I'll be considering what I would do differently *if I could turn back time*.

In the chapters that follow, I'll delve deeply into the hearts and minds of these unforgettable patients as they grapple with loss, betrayal, anxiety, depression, substance abuse, and other symptoms of the human condition. Brian, for example, recognized his father's bloodshot eyes and familiar sneer with each glance in his own mirror, as his life spiraled out of control from drug and alcohol abuse (see Chapter 3). Claire was an aging Southern belle whose irritability scorched all those who crossed her path and worsened a depression that buried her in bed for days at a time (see Chapter 1). Mandy, a severely depressed young girl, was so terrified of closeness with me that she sat silently in my office during most of every session (see Chapter 6). Jen, a lonely and irritable middle-aged woman, battered me with criticism and hurled insults at me through seven long years of our work together (Chap-ter 5). And there are more.

As psychotherapists and psychoanalysts, our work is intimate, private, and often very isolating. There are no co-workers present to appreciate an interpre-tation that fills the room with the warm breeze of understanding, nor is there a supervisor listening to catch angry words before they leave our mouths. And there is no quality control for a job in which silence can be the ultimate abandonment or the most profound and empathic way to join a patient.

We focus on theory and technique at our conferences and in our case presentations, and we often share only the most successful highlights and outcomes of our work. We are much less inclined to write or speak about our role in the misattunements, ruptures, and enactments that are inevitable and, in fact, crucial parts of every treatment. We shy away from exploring our own pain, anger, shame, and regret, as if these are unfortunate distractions from our work rather than essential tools in our work.

My goal in this book is to offer an unflinching look at what went right and what went wrong in nine memorable treatments, bearing in mind that one's hindsight is never 20/20. I share my thoughts, feelings, triumphs, regrets, and heartbreaks of every shape and size. I focus on the ruptures and repairs between my patients and myself, including a special kind of rupture: the enactment. I explore how these experiences both helped and harmed my relationship with each patient and their treatment. And I discuss my conscious and unconscious missteps as I have come to understand them, because one cannot do this work with a full heart without missteps and the resulting moments of misattunement.

My Path

Growing up, "self-reflection" was about how my hair looked, and "how I was feeling" referred to whether my cold was better. Words such as "anxiety," "sadness," "shame," and "insecurity" were not part of my family's lexicon. There was little awareness that internal worlds existed, never mind an appreciation of the pain and turmoil that might simmer within them.

As the youngest of three, I was considered the unruly one in my family. I was cast in this role since my earliest memories of streaking bare-bottomed through a department store at three years of age and scaling neighborhood fences since I was five. In sixth grade, my parents laughed as I drained their wine glasses during dinners out and turned a blind eye when I sampled their liquor cabinet at home. By ninth grade, I was hosting parties at whichever neighbor's house I was babysitting, and by my junior year of high school, I was cutting more classes than I attended. My sister was the smart one, my brother was the creative one, and I was the wild one.

When I took my first psychology class during my senior year of high school, however, I was stopped in my tracks. My nearly comatose curiosity came back to life as I learned about the mysteries of the unconscious, the magic of dream interpretation, and the workings of the id, ego, and superego. Fears, needs, defenses, conflicts – it was as if a switch had been flipped on, and my world was suddenly in technicolor. By the time I learned about Erik Erikson's eight states of identity development, I was hooked.

I was never interested in the kind of knowing that involved history, literature, or debating politics. That kind of knowing was wielded like a sword by my intellectual father and academically competitive siblings. I was drawn to a different kind of knowing – intuiting what other people were feeling and sensing their longings and vulnerabilities. I could feel the pulse of their emotional jugular and anticipate the words they needed to hear to assuage their anger or ignite powerful feelings such as pride or shame. The world of psychology seemed to involve this kind of knowing, and for the first time, I wanted to learn more.

I can remember watching the character Dr. Gail Baldwin on the soap opera *General Hospital* during this time. She was a smart, strong, and subtly maternal psychologist who worked on the hospital's inpatient psychiatric unit and saw private patients in a beautifully decorated office. My first thought was that I could use one of those. This was followed by a wave of recognition that I wanted to *be* one of those.

My Approach

Today, as a clinical psychologist and relational psychoanalyst, I focus on my patient's inner world to help them build a stronger, more capable sense of self with improved self-esteem, more adaptive defenses, and a clearer understanding of their emotional needs. Together, we uncover the interpersonal patterns, roles, traumas, and expectations they carry from childhood into their current relationships. Through our focus on the vicissitudes of the therapeutic relationship, we revisit how they have suffered to get their most basic emotional needs met. With some patients, interpersonal conflicts are in the forefront. With others, their self-esteem and difficulty regulating their emotions require the lion's share of our therapeutic attention.

Before I share nine in-depth clinical stories and speculate what I would do differently "if I could turn back time," I will briefly discuss the psychoanalytic theories I have found helpful in my clinical work.

Self Psychology and Relational Self Psychology Theory

The self psychology school of psychoanalysis, originated by Heinz Kohut (Kohut, 1971, 1984), has helped me understand my own development and has influenced my approach to clinical work. I value how self psychology prioritizes empathy as the ideal way to learn about my patient's emotional world, create a safe and trusting therapeutic relationship, and serve as a critical agent of change. In sessions, I try to viscerally experience my patient's deepest feelings about themselves and others, including their sequestered hopes and fears and the emotional push and pull of their relationships. I try to see the world through my patient's eyes, think and feel as I imagine they do, and even physically inhabit the room as they seem to – especially when their experience is one of deep hurt or trauma. And I consider what each patient needs from me at any given moment and how these needs wax and wane over the course of our relationship. I want my patient to feel that we are on this expedition of change together and that their pain, both past and present, matters very much to me.

Kohut's theory evolved out of his psychoanalytic work with patients with narcissistic disorders. He described these patients as "characterized by a specific vulnerability: their self-esteem is unusually labile and, in particular, they are extremely sensitive to failures, disappointments, and slights" (Kohut, 1968; Kohut & Wolf, 1978, p. 413). Kohut believed that these disorders could not be adequately explained or effectively treated by the classical drive-and-defense model because the core disturbance in these patients was in their weakened self. This self was understood by Kohut as the center of the patient's inner world and the core of the personality.

Kohut believed that defects in the self were caused by the misattunement or neglect of early caregivers. He theorized that chronic misattunement derails the young child's emotional development, and if not addressed, these unmet needs lead to a weakened or defective self, unstable self-esteem, and problematic interpersonal relationships. To address these deficits, the therapist needs to provide specific experiences for their patient that are aimed at meeting these essential developmental needs and relational longings. Kohut termed these *selfobject* experiences and identified them as experiences that meet (1) the patient's need to be seen, appreciated, and even celebrated for their strengths and struggles (mirroring selfobject experiences), (2) their need for a safe harbor where emotional security, guidance, and strength are offered (idealized selfobject experiences), and (3) their need to feel a sense of likeness and belonging with another (twinship selfobject experiences). As the patient takes in the therapist's selfobject functions and experiences them as part of themselves, their feelings of self-cohesion and self-esteem are enhanced, and their emotional development is facilitated (Kohut, 1971, 1984; Strozier et al., 2022).

For example, Lydia, a young woman in an emotionally abusive marriage, needed my recognition and celebration of her strengths, her struggles, and manifestations of her uniqueness to develop the feelings of self-worth and self-confidence that she needed to stand up to her abusive husband (see Chapter 9). My patient Josh was an older adolescent who was battling anorexia. He relied on me as a strong, protective figure who could help him learn to regulate his intense emotions and develop greater self-understanding and feelings of self-worth (see Chapter 8). And there's my rageful patient Jen, who endured a lifetime of interpersonal conflict and desperately needed to feel that I both shared and understood her very human vulnerabilities of seething rage and profound loneliness (see Chapter 5). All my patients needed a wide range of emotional provisions in our relationship, each at different times and, often, in very different ways.

In my clinical work, I focus on what has been referred to as the *forward edge* as well as the *trailing edge* of my patient's behavior and communications. These concepts were originally discussed by Kohut in his supervision with Miller (1985) and were later expanded on by Tolpin (2002, 2009). The forward edge describes the adaptive strivings toward health hidden within my patient's symptomatic and often self-destructive behavior. The trailing edge refers to a person's internal conflicts and repetitive, toxic interpersonal patterns. I prioritize understanding with my patient that their symptomatic behavior often represents their best attempt to manage the internal conflicts, overwhelming emotions, and external stressors that have threatened their emotional survival.

This forward edge focus enhances my patient's self-understanding and lessens their feelings of shame. It enables me to access my empathy and manage my own emotional reactions so that I avoid falling into unproductive roles such as the lecturing parent or the enraged partner. And by focusing on the forward edge of my patient's behavior, I can more effectively highlight the risks and costs of their often-misguided attempts at coping and help them embrace more adaptive ways of managing their emotional and interpersonal world.

Jamie was a twenty-year-old heroin addict when our work together began (see Chapter 7). Throughout much of our four-year treatment, she would lie, steal, and abuse drugs and alcohol. Jamie was used to a lifetime of criticism and was no stranger to searing feelings of shame. Rather than highlight the disruptive and dangerous aspects of her behavior, she and I understood the adaptive function of her substance abuse and self-destructive behavior as her only means of managing her overwhelming emotions and telegraphing to others that her life was spinning out of control. We also understood the idealized selfobject functions that drugs served for her – calming her feelings of helplessness and inadequacy and helping her feel protected and powerful.

I appreciate the more recent influence of relational self psychology, with its enhanced focus on the emotional experience of both the patient and the analyst, including, as my clinical stories will demonstrate, the patient's emotional impact on the analyst. Magid and Shane (2017, 2018) have articulated many of the commonalities and important differences between traditional self psychology and relational self psychology. Perhaps most impactful, traditional self psychology describes a one-person psychology in which the therapist's role is to understand the patient's unmet developmental needs and provide selfobject functions for the patient to address these needs. Relational self psychology views the therapist as a full person in the therapeutic relationship – one who brings with them their own unmet needs and subjective experiences. In this view, empathic responsiveness embodies the therapist's understanding of the patient's pressing emotional needs as well as the therapist's own emotional history and subjective experience with the patient. As such, it is a two-person psychology that includes the intersubjective experiences of both the patient and the therapist, as well as the mutual impact of each on the other. The therapeutic relationship, therefore, offers the patient new and longed-for relational experiences and becomes a more powerful agent of change.

Another important difference involves relational self psychology's expansion of empathic responsiveness to include not only responses that reflect an understanding of the patient's inner world, but also those that consider the internal state of important others in the patient's world (Fosshage, 2003a). This is instrumental in helping patients begin to question their often-painful assumptions about the feelings and motivation of those close to them. It also helps them feel less alone and less ashamed of their own emotional struggles. For example, it was helpful to explore with my patient Daphne how she imagined her husband experienced her repeated pressure for him to make more money. Over the course of treatment, she began to understand that his shutting down emotionally was not his rejection of her. Rather, she became able to see this as his self-protective response to her triggering his feelings of inadequacy (see Chapter 4).

Steven Stern (2024) integrates forward- and trailing-edge ideology as it influences the kinds of relationships that could and should emerge in our treatments. Stern appreciates the importance and the inevitability of how painful interpersonal patterns from childhood are repeated with the analyst in the transference and terms this the *repeated relationship*. He highlights the value of creating a new kind of relationship, what he refers to as the *needed relationship* for optimal understanding, synchronicity, and closeness within each analytic partnership. The forward edge–focused, needed relationship is co-created with each patient and is continually recalibrated as the treatment progresses. The needed relationship includes a fusion of the patient's thwarted needs from childhood, their current interpersonal needs, and the constellation of feelings that the analyst experiences with the patient. Stern's focus on the uniqueness of each relationship and the need for the analyst's authentic responsiveness resonate deeply with the way I work.

Multiple Self-States Theory

The theory of multiple self-states (Bromberg, 1998, 2010; Davies, 1996, 1998) has impacted the way I understand my patients, their problematic behavior, and their resistance to change. This theory suggests that we all have different selves or self-states that live within us and that each self-state is motivated by its own unique needs and fears. The facets of the self that coalesce into discrete self-states may be dissociated as a result of subtle explicit or implicit parental reactions or because of more significant relational trauma. We may unconsciously propel different self-states to assume center stage in our conscious experience, shifting the very nature of how we feel about ourselves and others, and drastically influencing the choices that we make. Working with consciously sequestered versions of a self, compartmentalized aspects of a self, or, in extreme cases, dissociated selves has been considered essential to broadening and deepening a patient's emotional experience and self-understanding. I have found this focus to be instrumental in helping my patients overcome their self-destructive patterns and resistance to making and sustaining the changes they consciously seek.

The focus on multiple self-states is considered especially useful in the treatment of substance abuse and eating disorders (Burton, 2005; Director, 2002, 2005; Petrucelli, 2021). I have found the self-states approach extremely relevant to my work with substance abuse patients whose self-states are dominated by their strongly conflicting needs and fears. These patients may rely on drugs to escape one self-state and call forward another in an attempt to regulate their emotions, boost their self-esteem, or manage anticipated or existing interpersonal conflicts. For example, the timid, insecure patient may use drugs to bring out the version of them that bursts with social confidence and feels unburdened by the opinions of others. Similarly, the version of my patient that wrestles in session with intense feelings of shame and a determination to stay sober may take a back seat to the patient's drug-abusing self-state just hours later, when a conflict with their partner leaves them feeling angry and unappreciated.

Standard psychotherapy approaches and twelve-step programs encourage the disavowal of the thoughts, feelings, and experiences of the drug-abusing self-states. These approaches insist on abstinence and tend to focus exclusively on the damaging effects of the substance abuse. What these approaches fail to ask, however, is how the substance use is meeting the patient's needs and expressing what they otherwise have been unable to express. Relational theorists with a self-state focus seek to understand the adaptive purposes of drug use and the self-states that accompany this use. This approach examines how substance abuse and substance-abusing self-states help the patient manage their labile affect, severely low self-esteem, unstable sense of self, and dissociated relational longings. This approach incorporates Khantzian's self-medication theory (1987, 1995), in which the main purpose of excessive drug use is to help the patient tolerate and manage their painful emotions.

Director asserts, "the self that uses needs to be brought into the treatment project" (2005, p. 628). As the self-destructive self-state is invited into the treatment room, painful affects and hidden relational longings emerge within the therapeutic relationship. The clinician can then address this part of the patient and help them manage their emotions and interpersonal needs in a healthier way (Director, 2002, 2005).

For example, Brian's childhood was dominated by feelings of helplessness and shame. As a teen and young adult, these feelings were silenced by the development of his raging, drug-abusing self-state. It wasn't until we explored this self-state in session that we gained access to his hidden feelings of deep shame for not protecting his mother from his father's brutality. Once Brian could accept the helpless little boy in him and his own longing for protection, he began to turn to me for understanding and guidance. He was then gradually able to relinquish the protection and sense of control that drugs and alcohol had afforded him (see Chapter 3).

Misattunements, Ruptures, and Enactments

Today, I try to be as emotionally in sync with each patient as possible. I often imagine that my patient and I are taking a slow walk in the woods together as I listen closely to their stories. I hear their words and take in the implicit story that their manner communicates. I watch my patient's facial expressions and body language. I take note of the volume and pacing of their speech and any other clues that might help me understand their internal experience. I try to discern which version of them is showing up at any moment, why that self has emerged, and what they need most from me. While these challenges take center stage for me, I also notice my own thoughts, feelings, reveries, and bodily experiences to become aware of how my patient is affecting me and what is happening between us. With so much going on at once, it's natural that assumptions, hypotheses, and my own personal reactions abound.

Sometimes, I get it right, and my patient feels deeply understood. Other times, I get it wrong, and I face their stormy rage, the eerie quiet of their disappointment, or the hollow echo of their words of compliance.

Trying to know another person in this way sometimes means losing myself in messy emotional experiences that I don't fully understand in the moment. But by exploring the ruptures and enactments that occur within our relationship, I offer my patient a different kind of relational experience than they are used to – a relationship with someone who prioritizes their experience and can take an honest look at my own contribution to their pain.

Misattunements

The most benign of these potential missteps are *misattunements*. Attunement has been described by developmental theorists as the early caregiver's sensitive attention and timely provisions in response to their infant's cues about their emotional and physical needs (Stern, 1985; Lachman & Beebe, 1993). Self psychology focuses on how an early caretaker's chronic misattunement, including their lack of synchronicity with and understanding of their child's needs and communications, can derail the child's emotional development (Kohut, 1971, 1984). Because of such misattunement, the very normal emotional needs of the infant and young child are not met. These young children may grow into adults who present with difficulty regulating their self-esteem, a lack of self-cohesion, and a bevy of unmet emotional needs and conflictual interpersonal relationships.

Consequences of the therapist's misattunement in therapy are similar to what happens in the mother–child interactions. The ruptures that misattunements cause may be brief and harmless, or they can derail the therapeutic relationship and require immediate repair. In extreme cases, the treatment may be damaged beyond repair. Whereas most patients are emotionally affected by misattunements, narcissistically vulnerable patients tend to be the most severely injured by them. One of my more egregious misattunements was my observation to my very narcissistically fragile patient Jen (see Chapter 5). I pointed out that she arrived very late to recent sessions and then experienced great difficulty ending when our time was up. This comment provoked intense feelings of shame and reactive feelings of rage as Jen's powerful need for and fear of closeness with me was highlighted.

Rupture and Repair

The concept of a *rupture* in treatment has come to mean virtually any occurrence within the patient–therapist relationship that threatens their crucial bond, including misattunements, dissociations, impasses, and enactments (Kohut, 1984; Fosshage, 2003c; Muran, 2019). Kohut (1971, 1984) believed that the therapist's *empathic failure* disrupts the essential selfobject tie between patient and therapist. He focused on the rupture/repair cycle as one of the most important mechanisms of change in psychotherapy. In this dynamic, change occurs via *transmuting internalization* as the patient repeatedly experiences and gradually internalizes the therapist's selfobject functions, strengthening and expanding the self in the process (Kohut, 1971; Kohut & Wolf, 1978).

More specifically, as the therapist nondefensively acknowledges and explores their role in the rupture (e.g., admitting to not understanding what the patient is saying or not responding empathically to the patient's pain, perhaps even responding aggressively), the patient gradually learns to internalize important cognitive and affective abilities of the therapist. The therapist's willingness to own their misattunement and question what it was like for the patient enables the patient to feel seen, understood, and worthy. When this rupture/repair cycle happens repeatedly in treatment, internal psychic structures develop that facilitate coping, communication, self-esteem maintenance, and the ability to trust.

The inevitable triggering and replaying of dysfunctional dynamics from the patient's early years – transference manifestations – have been understood as a frequent cause of ruptures in treatment (Fosshage, 2003b). Repairing these ruptures by understanding both participants' conscious and unconscious contributions to the conflict is considered key to both the patient and the therapist experiencing new relational possibilities. Similarly, Lachman and Beebe (1993) describe how the process of *dyadic regulation*, the influence that the patient and therapist have on each other during the repair cycle, is instrumental in the development of new interpersonal patterns and expectations.

In their extensive examination of the rupture/repair experience in psychotherapy, Muran and Eubanks (2020) focus on the intersubjective contributions of both patient and therapist involved in the rupture/repair dynamic and highlight the need for the therapist to model traits such as curiosity and humility in the repair process. These researchers developed the Alliance-Focused Training Protocol, the AFT (Eubanks-Carter et al., 2015; Muran & Eubanks, 2020; Muran et al., 2010) to train therapists to better manage ruptures in treatment, thereby improving patient retention and treatment outcome. More recently, Eubanks et al.'s (2023) book includes a collection of numerous papers and clinical studies about the rupture/repair process in a variety of treatment modalities including group therapy (Tasca and Marmarosh, Chapter 2) and couples and family therapy (Friedlander and Escudero, Chapter 3). In these chapters, common types of ruptures in each of these modalities are discussed, as are strategies for repair that are unique to each modality.

Some of the ruptures I describe in this book felt like "uh-oh" moments in which I longed to take back my words milliseconds after they had left my mouth. Other ruptures seemed more like the steady drum of benign interactions that built slowly and then suddenly took over the treatment room. In both cases, my patients and I struggled to find safer ground outside of the conflict where together, we could understand how and why one or both of us had been injured.

For example, I write about times in my work with Jamie, a twenty-year-old opiate addict (see Chapter 5), when I snapped like an angry parent in response to her life-threatening acting out and chronic lying. Jamie would then offer an insincere apology, emotionally shutting down in the face of my judgment and anger. As I understood my own feelings of anxiety and help-lessness that led to my angry parental reaction, I explored with Jamie how my response made her feel. I asked her if, in the future, I could tell her when her self-destructive behavior was making me feel particularly uncomfortable. Jamie warmed noticeably to my acknowledging my reaction and my willing-ness to share my own vulnerability with her. She playfully began to call me by her very anxious mother's first name when she sensed my anxiety or disap-proval, a tactic that helped me to immediately self-reflect and enabled us to experience a feeling of synchronicity that we had not previously shared.

Enactments

Enactments are powerful, unconsciously driven patient/therapist interactions that can be disruptive, healing, or both. Relational analysts (Aron, 2003; Atlas, 2020; Benjamin, 2010; Bromberg, 2003; Harris, 2002; Stern, D.B., 2004, 2013; Stern, S., 2016) describe enactments as interpersonal dramas that emerge between patient and therapist when unconscious issues from each of their inner worlds collide. In enactments, either member of the dyad may get emotionally pulled into the other's unique and often maladaptive relational patterns. As patient and therapist engage in and work through enactments together, each gains greater access to their own and the other's inner world.

Enactments offer the analyst a way to reach a patient's split-off self-states as their unconscious longings and expectations of others become activated in the here and now of the patient–therapist relationship (Benjamin, 2010). With some patients, enactments are the only way to access sequestered self-states and the intolerable affects that infuse them (Bromberg, 2006). For patients such as substance abusers, who often rely on action rather than words to express their pain, enactments represent nonverbal modes of communication that offer unparalleled access to dissociated feelings and self-states. In addi-tion to making these dissociated self-states available for conscious exploration, the working through of enactments enhances feelings of closeness and trust between patient and therapist (Gilhooley, 2011).

Donnel Stern (2004), a member of the Boston Change Process Study Group, suggests that enactments can take the form of "now moments" – spon-taneous, affectively charged, and unpredictable moments between patient and therapist. These kinds of occurrences, if authentically responded to by the analyst, may become "moments of meeting" that catalyze significant intra-psychic and relational change (Boston Process Change Study Group, 2010). These moments are emotionally laden lived experiences between patient and therapist and don't necessarily involve making the unconscious or dissociated available for verbal exploration.

As you will read, such a moment occurs in Chapter 4, when I leap across my office to look at the painting on my wall that my patient Nicki, a severely depressed adolescent, was referencing. As my otherwise lethargic patient jumped up to meet me at the painting, my dissociated wish to bring her back to life fused with her desperate longing for a mother who was "alive." The result was a shocking turning point in our work together.

In-actments

Finally, I focus on what I call *in-actments* – instances that occur when my patient and I unconsciously collude to *not* know, *not* see, and *not* act, often at an important moment in my patient's life. I see an "*in*-actment" as a mutual, unconscious avoidance in the service of both the patient and the therapist's respective emotional needs and narcissistic vulnerabilities. For example, my patient Josh's longing to capture "the gleam in my eye" (see Chapter 8) colluded with my need to feel like the good mother/healing therapist whose hard work was helping Josh succeed academically. As a result of our "*in*-actment" to not see, not know, and, therefore, not take steps to prevent his freezing when confronted with an important academic challenge, Josh nearly blew up his chance to gain admission to his dream school.

As you will see in the clinical stories that fill this book, I experienced enactments and *in*-actments much like swimming in the ocean: sometimes, my patient and I were gently pushed or pulled by the emotional waves; sometimes, we were knocked off our feet. As old feelings and toxic patterns filled the treatment room, we often felt tossed about by forces we couldn't fully understand or control. But once back on dry land, we reflected on our experience together and had an opportunity to discover vulnerabilities and strengths we didn't know were there. And we had a chance to discover each other in a new way.

A Bit of Courage

Years ago, in another life, I used to play competitive tennis. I wasn't a country club player who took weekly lessons. I was a scrapper with a one-handed backhand, a two-handed backhand, and occasionally, a left-handed forehand instead of a backhand. I would dive across the court if it meant getting to the ball in time. I simply hated to lose. And I knew that when a match got close, the worst thing I could do was to play scared.

Similarly, we cannot work scared when doing intensive psychotherapy or psychoanalysis. Misattuned responses and clinical missteps are inevitable. We will be pulled into enactments with our patient if the emotional connection is a powerful one. Many of these experiences will shed light on important aspects of our patient's inner world and relational patterns that we could never quite put our finger on otherwise. Some of these inevitable experiences may be harmful, but I believe one of the biggest mistakes a therapist can make is to play scared – to be afraid to get close enough, to care enough, to let oneself go enough to risk getting swept away – to risk sometimes getting it wrong.

As we experience the dawn of AI, I question whether a perfectly attuned, insight- and empathy-dispensing therapy bot will do a better job than I or any other living, breathing clinician. I suggest, however, that it is our longing to heal, our wish to protect, and our very human emotional vulnerability that helps our patients connect with us, trust us, and have hope that we can help them in a truly meaningful way.

In the pages that follow, I share with you my challenges, my triumphs, and my missteps, misattunements, ruptures, enactments, *in*-actments, and the things that I simply wish I had done differently in nine memorable treatments. The clinical details in each story are as true to my recollection as possible, although the personal details about each patient are altered significantly to preserve their confidentiality and anonymity. In fact, several case studies represent a composite of two or more different cases. I will strive for accuracy and emotional honesty in the pages that follow, but I must warn you, when things cut deep or wander into sequestered areas, I may have limited success.

References

Aron, L. (2003). The paradoxical place of enactment in psychoanalysis: Introduction. *Psychoanalytic Dialogues*, 13: 623–631.

Atlas, G. (ed.). (2020). *When minds meet: The work of Lewis Aron*. Routledge.

Benjamin, J. (2010). Where's the gap and what's the difference? The relational view of intersubjectivity, multiple selves, and enactments. *Contemporary Psychoanalysis*, 46: 112–119.

Boston Process Change Study Group. (2010). *Change in psychotherapy: A unifying paradigm*. Norton Professional Books.

Bromberg, P. (1998). *Standing in the spaces: Essays on clinical process, trauma, and dissociation*. The Analytic Press.

Bromberg, P. (2003). One need not be a house to be haunted: On enactment, dissociation, and the dread of "not me" – A case study. *Psychoanalytic Dialogues*, 13: 689–709.

Bromberg, P. (2006). "Ev'ry time we say good-bye, I die a little . . . " Commentary on Holly Levenkron's "Love (and hate) with a proper stranger." *Psychoanalytic Inquiry*, 26: 182–201.

Bromberg, P. (2010). Minding the dissociative gap. *Contemporary Psychoanalysis*, 46: 19–31.

Burton, N. (2005). Finding the lost girls: Multiplicity and dissociation in the treatment of addiction. *Psychoanalytic Dialogues*, 15: 587–612.

Davies, J.M. (1996). Linking the "pre-analytic" with the postclassical: Integration, dissociation and the multiplicity of unconscious process. *Contemporary Psychoanalysis*, 32: 553–576.

Davies, J.M. (1998). Multiple perspectives on multiplicity. *Psychoanalytic Dialogues*, 8: 195–206.

Director, L. (2002). The value of relational psychoanalysis in the treatment of chronic drug and alcohol use. *Psychoanalytic Dialogues*, 12: 551–579.

Director, L. (2005). Encounters with omnipotence in the psychoanalysis of substance users. *Psychoanalytic Dialogues*, 15(4): 567–586.

Eubanks, C., Samstag, L., & Muran, J.C. (2023). *Ruptures and repair in psychotherapy. A critical process for change*. American Psychological Association.

Eubanks-Carter, C., Muran, J.C., & Safran, J.D. (2015). Alliance-focused training. *Psychotherapy*, 52(2), 169–173.

Fosshage, J.L. (2003a). Contextualizing self psychology and relational psychoanalysis: Bi-directional influence and proposed synthesis. *Contemporary Psychoanalysis*, 39: 411–448.

Fosshage, J.L. (2003b). Fundamental pathways to change: Illuminating old and creating new relational experience. *International Forum for Psychoanalysis*, 12: 244–251.

Fosshage, J.L. (2003c). Some reflections on "what is a psychoanalytic relationship? and "how does it effectuate change?" *Psychoanalytic Perspectives*, 1: 45–53.

Gilhooley, D. (2011). Mistakes. *Psychoanalytic Psychology*, 28: 311–333.

Harris, A. (2002). Multiplicity as a form of enactment: Commentary on paper by Graham Bass. *Psychoanalytic Dialogues*, 12: 827–835.

Khantzian, E.J. (1987). A clinical perspective of the cause-consequence controversy in alcoholic and addictive suffering. *Journal of the American Academy of Psychoanalysis*, 15: 521–537.

Khantzian, E.J. (1995). Chapter 2: Self-regulation vulnerabilities in substance abusers: Treatment implications. *The Psychology and Treatment of Addictive Behavior*, 79: 17–41.

Kohut, H. (1968). The psychoanalytic treatment of narcissistic personality disorders: Outline of a systematic approach. In: *The search for the self: Selected writings of Heinz Kohut. 1950–1978*, vol. 1, P.H. Ornstein (ed.). International Universities Press, pp. 477–509.

Kohut, H. (1971). *The analysis of the self*. International Universities Press.

Kohut, H. (1984). *How does analysis cure?*, 2nd ed., A. Goldberg (ed.). University of Chicago Press.

Kohut, H., & Wolf, E.S. (1978). The disorders of the self and their treatment: An outline. *International Journal of Psychoanalysis*, 59: 413–425.

Lachman, F.M., & Beebe, B. (1993). Chapter 4. Interpretation in a developmental perspective. *Progress in Self Psychology*, 9: 45–52.

Magid, B., & Shane, E. (2017). Relational self psychology. *Psychoanalysis, Self and Context*, 12(1): 3–19.

Magid, B., & Shane, E. (2018). The restoration of the selfobject. *Psychoanalysis, Self and Context*, 913(3): 246–258.

Miller, J. (1985). How Kohut actually worked. In: *Progress in self psychology*, vol. 1, A. Goldberg (ed.). Guilford Press, pp. 13–30.

Muran, J.C. (2019). Confessions of a New York rupture researcher: In insider's guide and critique. *Psychotherapy Research*, 29(1): 1–14. https://doi.org/10.1080/10503307.2017.1413261

Muran, J.C., & Eubanks, C.F. (2020). *The therapist under pressure: Negotiating emotion, difference, and rupture*. American Psychological Association. https://doi.org/10.1037/0000182-000

Muran, J.C., Safran, J.D., & Eubanks-Carter, C. (2010). Developing therapist abilities to negotiate alliance ruptures. In: *The therapeutic alliance: An evidence-based guide to practice*, J.C. Muran & J.P. Barber (eds.). Guilford Press, pp. 320–340.

Petrucelli, J. (2021). Linking self-states in eating disordered patients: Multiplicity in multidisciplinary teams. *Psychoanalytic Dialogues*, 31: 205–213.

Stern, D.B. (2004). The eye sees itself: Dissociation, enactment, and the achievement of conflict. *Contemporary Psychoanalysis*, 40: 197–237.

Stern, D.B. (2013). Relational freedom and therapeutic action. *Journal of the American Psychoanalytic Association*, 61: 227–255.

Stern, D.N. (1985). *The interpersonal world of the human infant: A view from psychoanalysis and developmental psychology*. Basic Books.

Stern, S. (2016). Enactments in psychoanalysis: Therapeutic benefits. *Psychodynamic Psychotherapy*, 44(2): 281–303.

Stern, S. (2024). Breathing together: Needed relationships and complex selfobjects. *Psychoanalysis, Self and Context*, 19: 274–285.

Strozier, C.B., Pinteris, K., Kelley, K., & Cher, D. (2022). *The new world of self: Heinz Kohut's transformation of psychoanalysis and psychotherapy*. Oxford University Press.

Tolpin, M. (2002). Doing psychoanalysis of normal development: Forward edge transferences. *Progress in Self Psychology*, 18: 167–190.

Tolpin, M. (2009). A new direction for psychoanalysis: In search of a transference of health. *International Journey of Self Psychology*, 4: 31–43.

1   Waiting for Someone to Miss Me

Introduction

The story of Claire's life and death is one that will haunt me forever. It is a therapist's worst nightmare to have a patient commit suicide on their watch. While I believe I did everything in my power to help Claire manage her depression, see herself with fresh eyes, and feel deeply understood and valued in our relationship, in the end, she still chose the respite of death. This stark fact leaves me questioning my role in Claire's devastating final choice and whether there was more that I could have done to help her want to keep living.

Ours was a ten-month treatment in which I constantly monitored the pulse of the therapeutic relationship. I was always concerned that Claire's fear of closeness left her increasingly vulnerable as she began to feel more attached to me. In this story, I discuss how I understood the shifting emotional tides in Claire and in myself and how I tried to work with Claire's underlying feelings of rage and envy. I examine Claire's emotional reactions to me and my concern that she couldn't tolerate ruptures in our relationship so early in our work together. In this chapter as in the others, we will look at what went right and what could have and perhaps should have been handled differently.

Waiting for Someone to Miss Me

"I'm sorry, Dr. Feldman, Claire has killed herself. The police found her body last night. An overdose. . . ." Claire's older sister broke in midsentence, as if no further words were necessary. Simone, a strong, successful woman in her early fifties, delivered the news in clipped sentences. "Our family is grateful for the care you showed her. I'm sorry," she added in her rush to get off the phone.

I stood motionless in front of a rack of vegan leather pants in a neighborhood clothing store. "My patient killed herself," I whispered numbly to my twenty-year-old daughter. Suddenly, she was hugging me. I felt the abrupt shutdown of my emotions, like an amusement park ride that stopped in midair to address an emergency. All feelings off the ride; this one's going to be down for a while.

DOI: 10.4324/9781003543343-2

When the shock slowly began to wear off, the questions and seeds of self-condemnation began to take root in my mind. Why didn't I know what Claire was planning? What could I have done to prevent this tragedy? These subtle accusations were followed by my heartfelt question of whether it was my mandate or even my right to insist that Claire soldier on when her life was one of unending misery.

I knew of Claire's lifelong thoughts of suicide and desperate longing for relief from her bottomless sadness, but her final choice was still a shock to me. I wondered why she had never attempted this before despite decades of severe depression and painful isolation. What had Claire been waiting for? She seemed to hold onto a child's hope that one day, someone would truly see her, understand her, and perhaps even value her. In our ten months of work together, I hoped that I could be that someone for Claire.

Claire was the younger of two daughters and always felt like the wrong kind of little girl for her wealthy Southern family. Too loud, too active, and too hungry for attention, she felt defenseless against her mother's insistence on academic success and "proper" social behavior. Claire was the little girl who tracked mud on the white living room rug. She was the child who was constantly hushed at the dinner table. The more she clamored to be heard, the faster and more furiously the adults in her world shut her down.

As a teenager, auburn-haired, hazel-eyed Claire was strikingly beautiful. While she first appeared wild and carefree, the truth was in her eyes. Her desperate stare told the story of an aching loneliness. By high school, Claire's cutting classes, conflict with her peers, and excessive fondness for Jack Daniels prompted her parents to send her to an all-girls Catholic school. Here too, she felt too loud, too active, and too messy for the refined and very disciplined tastes of others. Both at school and at home, she was an outsider, face pressed against the glass and fists pounding on it, raging because no one would let her in.

Claire had just turned forty-seven when I met her. She had a long history of volatile relationships, self-medicating with pills, and severe bouts of depression. While she entertained frequent thoughts of suicide throughout her life and had a long history of impulsive behavior and poor judgment, she had never actively tried to hurt herself. More recently, Claire also began to have panic attacks, which made even going to the grocery store an ordeal. After years of refusing medication, she finally acquiesced and was on a combination of mood-stabilizing and antidepressant medications. Claire was encouraged by the relief that these pills gave her, so when her psychiatrist recommended that she speak to a therapist, she agreed to give it a try.

I greeted Claire in the waiting room for our first session and was flooded with a rush of visual stimulation. Her hair was a bright red, her blouse a floral mix of orange and yellows, and her lipstick was the brightest pink. She wore jeans with old red cowboy boots, an outfit seemingly chosen to awaken and interest a disinterested world.

Claire strode into my office with her shoulders back and her head held high in a purposeful manner that felt exhausting to me. She examined me carefully before settling into the large leather armchair and training her eyes on mine. Claire seemed to be assessing the bright colors of my own casual attire as well as my willingness to hold her intense gaze. We were each intrigued by the other.

In our first session, Claire spoke at length about her longstanding battle with depression. She attributed her years of emotional agony to decades of criticism by her parents, exclusion by her peers, and rejection by men. As she spoke, I felt the crushing sadness that had been her constant companion and had the sense that this outwardly colorful and challenging woman was more alone than anyone I had ever met.

Toward the end of the session, I suggested that we meet twice weekly. Claire shifted uncomfortably in her seat and said, "I would love to meet with you that much, I really would. I just don't know what we would talk about. My life isn't that interesting anymore. It was once, but it isn't anymore."

I felt her longing for connection silently battle her terror of being found lacking and turned away. And I wondered if she sensed the rage and envy boiling inside her and unconsciously worried that our work together might unleash these demons.

Assessing Claire's ability to consider conflict in a deeper way, I asked, "Are you afraid that you'll disappoint me – that if you're not interesting enough, I might not want to meet with you at all?"

Claire responded, "I don't know. You seem very nice. I just don't want to waste your time."

I felt torn between staying with her fear of rejection and presenting myself as someone who could offer her a modicum of hope. I sensed that her dread of rejection was coming alive in the room, and I was concerned that if I pushed too hard, she might feel too vulnerable in our very first session. I settled for reassuring the hopeful little girl inside of her and said, "Let's give it a try. I'm looking forward to getting to know you." She agreed.

As Claire left my office, I noted my own silent battle. This was a woman that I very much wanted to help, but her lifetime of suffering left me with an uneasy feeling deep in my core. I wonder if I sensed, so early in our work together, that the desolation of Claire's emotional world might prove unbearable for me and that I might fall short of giving her the kind of help she so desperately needed.

In the next few sessions, Claire shared detailed stories about the parents of her childhood, and I quickly understood how the seeds of mistrust and self-hate had been planted in her earliest years. Her mother was a self-involved, easily irritated woman whose time was spent attending to her perfectly manicured nails, youthful hairdo, and daily 3 p.m. doubles game at the club. She was constantly bothered by Claire, who seemed to embody a raw neediness and lack of self-control that her mother despised. In the face of her mother's relentless criticism, Claire got tattoos and piercings. She hopped on the back of motorcycles and into the back seats of cars with boys who promised little beyond a few moments of attention and excitement.

Claire described her father as another disappointment. He was a successful lawyer who worked sixteen-hour days and was too wrapped up in his golf game to do more than glance in his younger daughter's direction. While Claire's father seemed proud of her sister's popularity, he bristled at the conflict and drama that filled Claire's relationships, both at home and at school.

I winced as I imagined growing up with these cold, self-involved parents. I understood that, at times, I would be experienced as like them and readied myself to absorb Claire's feelings of longing and fury. I felt the need to validate her pain and anger and appreciate with her the hidden signs of her resilience. I believed that supporting Claire's tendrils of strength and health in the face of growing up with these self-absorbed, critical parents would be an important facet of our work together.

As the treatment progressed, I learned that Claire lived alone in a two-bedroom apartment that was filled with the vestiges of her failed marriage and the four-bedroom suburban home she was forced to give up. Her ex-husband's infidelity was a tragic disappointment, made worse by his rejection when she begged him to give their marriage a second chance. "That must have been awful," I offered, and after a long pause, I asked, "Can you tell me more about your marriage?"

"I don't know. I wasn't young enough or pretty enough for him anymore. I promised him that I would take better care of myself – I'd get up earlier and start exercising again. I'd clean the house and drink less. Shit, I even promised that I'd have sex with him more. But I couldn't make myself thirty again, and that's what mattered to Steven," Claire explained definitively.

I made a mental note of Claire's focus on her appearance and sexual availability as the reasons for her husband's infidelity and the failure of their marriage. I strongly sensed that Claire was not ready for me to challenge this idea. Instead, we talked about the devastation of this abandonment, which was magnified a hundredfold when he married his secretary just months after their divorce. As Claire shared this last detail, she spat, "She wasn't even prettier than me, just younger," and then venomously added, "Fuck them both. I hope they die."

Claire had no friends of her own and little contact with her sister, so when her marriage ended, she was very much alone. She related to others with an unfortunate blend of intrusiveness and severe irritability. Her frequent arguing with patrons at the beauty salon where she answered phones routinely jeopardized her job. And her combative behavior at the neighborhood bar left her feeling like an outsider among outsiders. Tragically, though Claire was tormented by her loneliness and isolation, she was utterly disdainful of the few equally lost souls who were eager to engage with her.

As Claire settled into our work together, she began to enjoy having an interested audience of one. She gradually invited me deeper into her emotional world, offering stories of lost opportunities and unfair rejections. As

I tried to temper her feelings of self-hate and resentment with validation and understanding, Claire warmed to me. In these moments, I felt like the mother she had longed for. One could empathize with her pain and embrace her idiosyncrasies, rather than despise and ridicule her for them.

I began to understand Claire's deep-seated belief that she was damaged and unlovable. She seemed to see herself like an old peacock, one who had lost the bulk of her feathers and was a sad and slightly frightening sight. Because her attractiveness was all that she used to feel was redeeming about her, Claire now believed that she had nothing to offer the outside world.

Claire's view of other people was polarized. Those who were seen as damaged, like herself, were dismissed without a second thought. She disdainfully referred to them as "losers" and felt that they were "of no use to me." Claire looked up to those with partners and families with a mixture of envy and admiration but felt certain they were also selfish and cruel – rejectors lying in wait should she give them the opportunity to hurt her. As I saw how these perceptions defined her expectation of others, I understood that the possibility of relationships was smothered in dread and all but doomed to fail. Again, I considered that my relationship with Claire would be the linchpin of our work together and felt the need to proceed carefully.

I paid close attention to the emotional shifts in our relationship. Claire seemed to fear that, like her mother, I would respond to her neediness or anger by dismissing her. She often smothered me with ingratiating compliments, consciously offered to win my favor, unconsciously designed to manage her underlying feelings of rage and envy. I found these moments particularly trying but feared that exploring them with Claire might deal a humiliating blow to her fragile ego and our tenuous bond. At this time, fostering her self-esteem and building her trust in me as an empathic, protective figure took priority over helping her gain insight into her unconscious motivation and problematic interpersonal patterns.

In hindsight, I wonder if I should have spoken with Claire more directly about her emerging feelings for me and more actively encouraged her to voice her negative and positive feelings, including those of longing, envy, and resentment. I focused on helping her feel understood and valued in our relationship, but I wonder if she felt the need to internalize more painful and aggressive feelings to maintain my acceptance and protect our relationship. I question whether my need to feel like a good mother with Claire eclipsed my recognition of her need to be a rageful child with me.

Claire began most sessions in a fawning manner that triggered sharp feelings of intrusion and annoyance in me. "Good morning, Dr. Feldman. Did you have a good weekend? You look so nice today. I love your shoes. You always have the best shoes," Claire said one day as she strode into the room. Her eyes were hungry and searching, and while she was smiling, I could feel the envy oozing from the corners of her words. As the session unfolded, my quiet attention steadied her, and she began to speak about her life and her loneliness in a truly touching way. I could see her edges soften as her defenses relaxed, and I felt a genuine warmth between us emerge. This was a common pattern in our sessions, and in these moments, I felt a closeness to Claire.

At other times, Claire raged about the "bitches" at her job, the "pieces of shit" living in her apartment building, or the "lowlifes" at the neighborhood bar. At these times, it was clear to me that I was there to witness and validate her suffering but not to question her perceptions or critique her interactions with others.

When the toxic bitterness that filled her emotional world infused the treatment room, I sometimes struggled just to breathe. Again, I wonder if I should have taken on her anger more directly and helped her understand how her verbal snipes and tirades impacted those around her. Highlighting her rage and processing it with her might have enabled Claire to eventually metabolize her own anger rather than continue to turn it against herself or spew it at others with the slightest provocation. Instead, I chose to focus on helping her understand the old wound that had been inflamed and better manage her reactivity.

Claire's more severe depressive episodes led her to miss work and spend endless days in bed. Despite this, she rarely missed a session with me and always found the energy to talk about the demoralizing life experiences that were derailing her. During one session, she dared to give voice to her envy. Claire spoke defeatedly as she described the emptiness of her weekend – watching old movies and searching through magazines for clothes she could no longer afford to buy. She then looked up at me and said nothing for several minutes. After what felt like an eternity, I asked, "What are you thinking?"

"I'm wishing I was you," Claire responded with a melancholy voice and piercing stare that left me speechless.

When I slowly regained my ability to speak, I quietly said, "Tell me more."

"Oh, Dr. Feldman," she sighed, "to be you. To have a home and a family and a dog and a life. To be you."

Overwhelmed by this surge of longing and envy, I found myself searching for a sliver of consolation that Claire's world could hold for her. I felt the weight of her hopelessness and my own fear that she might always feel this way. Finally, to escape the raw pain that filled the room, I asked, "Tell me about the life you would want. Paint me a picture."

Claire described the small rescue dog she longed to have, one who would love her unconditionally and carry her through the worst of her depression. We talked about this little bundle of hope and how each would rescue the other. "Maybe one day," Claire said, "when I have more money and more energy. Right now, I can barely take care of myself."

Again, I felt torn between addressing Claire's envy and prioritizing her feelings of idealization and safety with me. Exploring her envy risked triggering her intense feelings of shame, and I worried it would have caused a rupture in our young relationship that she was unable to tolerate. On the other hand, my understanding and normalizing these excruciating feelings with Claire might have lessened them. I told myself that once I felt Claire could tolerate talking about her intensely ambivalent feelings toward me, we could use our relationship to work through the difficult and painful feelings that had infused her past close relationships.

In this conversation as in others, I chose to stay with Claire's experience, seeking to witness and hold if not lessen her pain. I told myself that one day I would share with her the sadness that her loneliness stirred in me. One day, I would talk with her about the pain and frustration I felt as I watched her create and recreate her emotional exile from an unforgiving world. While I knew in my heart that "one day" was a long way away, I had no idea that there were only moments left on our clock.

Claire talked about her worsening depression over the holiday season shortly before her death. I offered her additional sessions, contracted with her regarding her safety, and arranged family sessions with her sister to improve communication between them. "Please call me or text me if you need to talk," I all but pleaded in our last session before the long Christmas weekend. Despite my efforts to keep her tethered to our relationship, I worried that Claire was being pulled away by the relentless force of her depression. I also felt a gnawing sense of guilt as I anticipated the warmth of my upcoming holiday and imagined the emptiness of hers.

Claire made it through the holiday and was seemingly on track with both her work and our sessions together. She burst into the session after Christmas and asked in a forced, upbeat voice, "How were your holidays, Dr. Feldman? Did you have a wonderful time with family?"

I knew that all potential answers to these questions were fraught with danger, but refusing to engage on a personal level seemed the most potentially rejecting. "Not bad," I responded. "Lots of traffic and too much food. But I've been thinking about you and how this past week has been for you."

Claire gave me a sad smile and answered, "Well, not as good as yours, I'm sure. My cousin Betty invited me over for Christmas. A pity invite, you know. She waited until three days before. She lives all the way in Central Jersey. My sister and her family go there every year. I just couldn't. I blamed it on the long drive, but I don't have the money to buy everyone presents. It just would have made me feel worse. My sister sent me a cooked ham and some kind of fancy potatoes. They weren't very good, of course, but I didn't even send her or her kids a card."

"Sounds hard. How did you make it through the holiday?" I asked, truly wondering how she survived the isolation and her overwhelming feelings of inadequacy.

"I did what I always do," she said matter-of-factly. "I took a few pills and went to sleep."

My heart hurt for Claire as I considered this habit of sleeping through special days and the deep pain that necessitated this. I was so uncomfortable with the depth of her despair and longed to brainstorm with her about how she could remedy her loneliness. Again, I sensed that Claire was not ready for this and that isolation was more tolerable than the feelings of self-loathing and resentment that even casual relationships stirred in her. Claire had survived her forty-seventh Christmas. She was back at work and back in my office, soaking up my interest in her and sharing her daily struggles. It wasn't until her car broke down, two weeks into February, that her severe depression once again reared its head.

Car trouble seemed to highlight the desperation of Claire's situation. Her alimony barely covered her rent, and her job at the beauty salon offered little cushion for the rest of her bills. In addition to the financial pressure, there was no willing partner or friend to help her get from place to place. Though terribly stressful, none of this was new for Claire. Again, I quieted my need to "do something" and consoled myself with the idea that at least now, she had me to confide in and validate how overwhelming all of this was for her.

Claire and I had a typical session on the third Monday in February. She talked about her cousin Betty and reminisced about how the two of them used to sneak off to smoke pot as teenagers to endure endless family get-togethers. Betty was homely, Claire explained, and not particularly interesting. She added resentfully that Betty was certainly doing well for herself now, with a husband, two kids, and a well-paying job as a paralegal.

Claire lamented that the beauty of her own youth had gotten her exactly nowhere and that at forty-seven, she no longer had that anymore. We talked about how dull she found her job at the beauty salon but cited her need for money as the reason she kept a job "so far beneath me." So when Claire left a message on Wednesday saying that the salon needed her to work on Thursday and she couldn't make our session, I didn't think much of it. She ended her message with, "I'll see you Monday." But Claire's Monday session never came.

More than a year since her death, I am held in place by the idea that Claire and I shared her battle, and without a word, seemingly without a sign, she left. I have often asked myself how I failed Claire and what accounts for the sinking feeling deep in my gut when I think of her. When all is very quiet, my heart whispers, "You didn't love her. Sometimes, you struggled to even like her."

As I think back on our work together, I wonder if I should have shared more of my own thoughts and feelings with Claire. Given her extreme sensitivity, I worried that direct feedback would have been experienced as criticism. Sharing my more positive feelings toward her might have activated her overwhelming longing for admiration and dread of rejection. I was also concerned that by inserting my feelings into the treatment room, I would be experienced as the self-involved, narcissistic mother of her childhood. Yet not doing so and indulging my own preference for emotional privacy may have cast me in that cold and uncaring role just the same.

I realize that by avoiding being experienced as the self-serving parent of her past, I was also avoiding conflict and rupture with Claire. While my reticence to work through her rage may have been wise in the early stages of our work, it nonetheless denied Claire the opportunity to work through her anger or to experience emotional repair within a close relationship.

I questioned why I didn't see her suicide coming. Had I missed the hesitation in her response or a downward glance when I asked about any thoughts of hurting herself? Did I stop asking pointed questions about her safety and her mood earlier than I should have? Had I exhaled too soon after the holidays and focused too much on her resilience? While I knew that patients were at a higher risk for self-harm as they came out of a severe depressive episode (and following holidays), Claire seemed actively engaged in our sessions and was talking about looking forward to the warmer weather, when she could be outside more and take long walks on a nearby boardwalk.

Claire's decision to end her life did not strike me as an impulsive response to an emotional blow or the last treacherous assault of her severe depression. Rather, I believe that it was a gradual wearing away of her will to live and desire to push through even one more lonely and meaningless day. I think she had simply had enough pain.

Finally, I've wondered if Claire felt unable to leave this world saddled with the aching fear that no one would miss her, or worse still, that no one would notice she was gone. Claire knew that I would notice her absence. I think she dared to hope that I would care deeply that she was gone. For better and certainly for worse, I believe Claire was waiting to have someone in her life who would miss her. By being this someone, perhaps I unwittingly gave her the peace of mind to finally let go.

If I Could Turn Back Time

Though it almost feels foolish to say so, if I could turn back time, I would not have handled Claire's suicidality differently. I offered her additional sessions and made myself available by phone and by text in between sessions. I discussed my concerns with Claire, and I contracted with her regarding her safety during the times she seemed most vulnerable. And I brought her sister in for a family session and consulted frequently with her psychiatrist. While I raised the question of hospitalization with Claire, she adamantly refused, and I respected her wishes. Claire was severely depressed, but this was not a new experience for her. She was clear-minded, and I imagine she felt some relief with her decision to end her life. And while I grieve her final, awful choice, I still believe that it was her choice to make.

As I consider the countless clinical decisions I made in my work with Claire, certain choices stand out for me. Given her emotional fragility and long history of interpersonal conflict and rejection, I prioritized creating and maintaining a safe and trusting relationship with her during our first year of treatment. If I could turn back time, I would keep a careful eye on the therapeutic bond, but I would also actively encourage Claire to share her intense feelings of anger and envy with me more freely, especially those directed toward me. Encouraging and embracing Claire's more uncomfortable and shameful feelings might have neutralized some of the toxicity of her internal world, normalized her experience of intense envy and rage, and helped her learn to manage both within the context of a close relationship. By talking through any disruptions in our relationship that might have been triggered, I could have modeled tolerating intense affect, owned my misattunement, and shown her that we both possess the ability to address and repair conflicts, misunderstandings, and disappointments in our relationship.

In hindsight, I wish I had highlighted Claire's resilience more – her hidden strength that kept her clinging to life during her painful adult years. Placing more emphasis on the emotional grit that enabled her to survive severe depression and devastating loneliness might have offered her the mirroring and validation that she craved and bolstered her desperately low self-esteem.

I was concerned that sharing my own experience with Claire might have felt like a repetition with her narcissistic mother in which Claire's needs always took a back seat to her mother's feelings and wishes. Looking back, I wonder if judiciously sharing my feelings of warmth and connection with Claire might have enhanced her self-esteem and assuaged her anxiety/terror around attachment. Similarly, sharing my deep feelings of sadness and demoralization in the face of her longstanding emotional pain might have provided the validation she needed and sense of likeness with another, or twinship experience, that she longed for.

Finally, as I became concerned about her worsening depression and the possibility of her self-harm, I wish that I had talked more with Claire about what her death would have meant to me. While it was difficult for her to tolerate seeing me as a separate person with my own strong feelings, I think telling her how deeply sad and upset I would have been if she were to kill herself might have made her feel truly important to another person.

2   Forever and a Moment

Introduction

One of the inspirations for this book was my work with Nicki. We had an amalgam of intense emotional experiences – her despair, my confusion, our similar but different feelings of helplessness, and her miraculous turnaround, all of which added to the power of our connection and made this a unique treatment. Perhaps more than anything, her love for her mother resonated deeply with me, both triggering my raw feelings of anxiety about my own aging mother and my deep admiration for her commitment to stay by her mother's side.

It took forever and it took a moment for Nicki to lose her mother and take a leap of faith with me. On a warm July afternoon, Nicki and I shared a moment in the middle of what seemed like an endless treatment that had been unable to halt her painful decline. This moment was an electric product of desperation – mine and hers – a "moment of meeting" (Boston Change Process Study Group, 2010) that hung in the air between us. I believe in my bones that it was this moment, ushered in by a break in the frame, that pulled Nicki over the invisible line between despair and hope.

"Forever and a Moment" is Nicki's story of survival and the story of the transformational power of a single moment in time. And it is the story of our years of work together that eventually made the magic of this moment between us possible.

Forever and a Moment

Nicki began treatment as an otherwise typical eighth grader who suddenly refused to leave home for school or discuss the reasons for this change in her behavior. In our first session, I met an extremely bright and beautiful fourteen-year-old girl who talked easily about her life with her stay-at-home mom and hardworking accountant father. Nicki described being from a traditional Jewish family, where her mother was responsible for every aspect of her and her younger sister's lives and her quiet father could be counted on for special outings on the weekends. She spent a great deal of time with her aunts

DOI: 10.4324/9781003543343-3

and female cousins, especially after temple. This unique group of women, young and old, was an important part of Nicki's day-to-day life throughout her childhood.

Nicki spoke in detail about her frequent shopping trips with her mother and their love of baking together. She spoke with relish about her Saturday-morning walks on the beach with her father, even on snow-filled winter mornings. Her older sister was annoying, and Nicki offered examples of how the two bickered daily, as any self-respecting siblings might. Her mother made pastries that friends and family raved about, her father led temple events, and they often hosted family and close friends in their home. Life was warm and good.

Early in treatment, a pattern emerged in our sessions. Nicki would tell me a long and colorful story, and I would be her appreciative audience. During one session, she talked at length about a weekend trip to the outlets with her mother. She recounted with amusement her mother's insistence on going to yet another store in search of the perfect gift for her aunt's birthday. In another session, she described helping her father with a carpentry project in their garage. She beamed as she remembered her father's proud smile when he admired the new shelves that he and Nicki had just installed. I longed to bask in these wholesome and heartwarming stories with her but always felt compelled to address the elephant in the room, the weekday battles around Nicki's refusal to go to school.

When Nicki talked about her shopping trip with her mom, I somewhat awkwardly said, "Sounds like quite the weekend. You guys seem to have a wonderful time together." After a long pause, I probed, "Nicki, can we talk about during the week? Can you take me through Monday morning, when it was time to go to school?"

Nicki's face dropped, and the shrug of her shoulders was now the only communication offered. As silence filled the room, my anxious brain began to calculate. How much quiet gave her the space to struggle without making her feel like she was disappointing me or I was angry with her for her silence?

As I felt the tipping point approaching, I said, "It seems so hard to put what's going on into words, even for someone who is as good with words as you. Can you help me understand?"

And with my plea for connection, Nicki looked down again, seemingly to consider her options. After a few moments of reflection, she looked up and met my gaze. Resuming our dance, Nicki deluged me with the details of her sister Rachel's weekend, including Rachel's search for the perfect prom dress that delayed their Sunday-night brisket dinner.

Nicki was able to talk about how she used to love being in school. She described dependably earning an A in almost all her classes. She would sit, head together with her two best friends, giggling and planning their weekend activities, as their teacher went over the homework that the three had easily completed. What Nicki couldn't put into words was why attending school suddenly felt unbearable. She and her mother had screaming fights when

Nicki defiantly refused to leave the house each morning. Her mother followed her from room to room, begging her to explain what was bothering her. On the rare day that her mother could drag her to school, Nicki spent silent hours in the guidance office. At these times, she was unwilling to walk into the classroom and was unable to discuss her struggle. School officials threatened her, her parents pleaded with her, and I tried desperately to understand this sudden self-imprisonment.

By the tenth grade, Nicki was deemed unmanageable by the public school system and was sent to a therapeutic day school, where she was promptly placed on antidepressant medication.

These measures had little effect, and Nicki became increasingly agitated and depressed. Feet planted squarely on the floor, she would read, cook, and clean at home but refused to go to school and only rarely agreed to go out with her cousins or friends. Despite this decline, Nicki never missed a session, showing up even on her darkest days.

Now sixteen, Nicki would come to sessions with mismatched clothes and unbrushed hair. She would hurry through the halls of reality with me, swatting away my weekly probes about school and home. Finally, she would settle in to tell me one of her favorite children's stories. She told me stories of a velveteen rabbit who longed to feel real and a lima bean–colored little girl who dared to be different. She bathed in moments of pleasure as she shared stories of shapeshifters and fairies from faraway worlds that she created during her long stretches of solitude in her bedroom. The telling of these stories enlivened Nicki, and she was particularly attuned to the subtle signs of my enjoyment. Nicki's stories had become a kind of offering, her attempt to be a good mother to both of us through this long, terrible time.

Nicki's stories were her form of play in our analytic space. Even at her lowest, Nicki clung tenaciously to her ability to play. I would later understand that this play was her salvation during endless hours alone in her home, guarding a mother whose body remained but whose mind was quietly disappearing. The play filled the "forever" of our work together and allowed Nicki to experience me as an attuned, admiring mother who could appreciate her ability to create in the face of deadness and despair.

My inability to get past Nicki's formidable defenses and understand the reasons for her school refusal was making me feel both frustrated and helpless. For me, the play felt like something I could engage in. Like a light through the fog of ineptness that hung over me, I followed Nicki's lead. It kept me emotionally tethered to her as we sat in my office, her depression deepening and her world falling apart. Nicki was uninterested in my questions about her feelings or her moods, and she routinely dismissed my concerns. Her stories became our lifeline: it was our connection with each other and my conduit to the part of Nicki that continued to grow despite the misery of her daily life.

I listened carefully to the nuances of Nicki's self-protective storytelling and tried to find an inroad to the corner of her mind that was forcibly shutting down contact with much of the outside world. I followed each story as if it were a treasure map, searching for clues to the deeper story it might tell – but to no avail. My frustration grew, but so did my appreciation of Nicki's storytelling and the deep, warm connection I felt with her during these moments.

My silent analysis of her stories yielded little, as did my questions about her school refusal. I felt terribly alone in my increasingly desperate attempts to understand what was causing this previously high-functioning teen to decompensate before my eyes. Was she being bullied or having issues with a teacher? Was she feeling an unmanageable pressure to perform? Or was an underlying psychotic process beginning to emerge? What I didn't think to ask was why it was so hard for her to leave her mother. My brief conversations with Nicki's mother at the start of each session never revealed any conflicts or concerns at home other than those around Nicki's school refusal.

Despite being in therapeutic day school, Nicki and I continued to meet until the end of her sophomore year, when she was forced to go to a residential school several hours away. I later learned that over the next two years, her mother began showing unmistakable signs of Alzheimer's, the disease that had been silently pecking away at her brain for years. What Nicki had unconsciously known was now part of her conscious reality, and she fought staying at the residential school with a renewed fierceness. Following her fourth episode of running away from the school and her second inpatient hospitalization for self-destructive and increasingly bizarre behavior, Nicki's desperately frustrated father allowed his daughter to come home. Within several weeks of her returning home to her rapidly deteriorating mother, Nicki's dad called me for an appointment.

With her sister away at college, Nicki and her father were her mother's only caretakers for the next two years. The shades were drawn for weeks on end, and day and night became indistinguishable. When she wasn't cleaning her mother or suffering through her disorganized tirades, Nicki would be alone in her room, safe in the imaginary world of books and her own stories.

My heart broke for Nicki as she became even more reclusive and disorganized. When her mother was finally placed in a facility, I hoped that being relieved of the overwhelming burden of caring for her would provide relief and opportunity for Nicki. Instead, depression and guilt continued to imprison her. She remained isolated in her home and, more days than not, spoke only to her father.

It was a Thursday in mid-July, two months after her mother was placed in a facility, when Nicki sulked into my office for her weekly session. Her beautiful auburn hair was straying in every direction. Her mismatched clothing screamed disorganization, and her soft brown eyes whispered despair. Uncharacteristically, Nicki wouldn't look at me or speak to me but inaudibly mumbled a few syllables in response to my questions.

Nicki half sat, half laid on my couch, looking more disheveled and depressed than I had ever seen her. After twenty minutes of long silences and monosyllabic responses, the air felt thick with hopelessness. I finally said,

"Feels like you are in a darker, lonelier place than I've seen you. Like in those dark mountains in that picture." And I nodded toward the painting on the far wall of my office.

Nicki slowly glanced up at the picture and quietly said, "Those aren't mountains, they are rocks with waves crashing on them."

Without thinking, I catapulted across the room to take a closer look at the picture.

Within half a second, Nicki met me across the room, and the two of us stood, elbow to elbow, in front of the picture.

"Show me where you see that," I asked.

What followed was an animated back-and-forth, comparing and contrasting our understanding of the picture. There was eye contact, there was dialogue, there was life.

Within a few moments, we sat down again, continued talking, and a more typical session ensued. I considered commenting on the moment we had just shared. Thankfully, I was silent. It was experience, not words, that rescued my patient from the emotional quicksand that was consuming her. Turning the beam of conscious reflection on that moment would have minimized it if not incinerated it.

The following week, Nicki walked into our session and shocked me with her announcement that she had registered for college. The next few weeks were filled with activity, including trips to Staples and meetings with her school advisor. One month later, Nicki started community college and insisted on taking a full course load. She got a volunteer job on campus and began to reconnect with her aunts and cousins. After seven long years of increasing anxiety, despair, and isolation, Nicki had suddenly, miraculously reengaged with the world of the living.

Fast forward nine months, and I lost my breath as I read a text from Nicki. "Hi Dr. Feldman. Just wanted you to know that I made Dean's List. Actually, I got straight A's."

My eyes filled with tears, and my heart soared with pride. I thought back on our moment in front of the picture in my office. For years, I felt that my only offering to Nicki was to bear witness to the tragedy that slowly unfolded before my eyes, forty-five minutes at a time. Then, suddenly, seemingly in a single moment, the dark waters of dysfunction parted, and a narrow path to the living world emerged.

This moment was not created by conscious thought, as my interpretations with Nicki often fell flat. It was not brought about by emotional attunement. My empathic responses seemed comforting but had little true impact. The moment seemed to be a result of the spontaneous connection between Nicki's despair and my own emotional turmoil around both my fear of losing my own mother and my inability to help my young patient. Made possible by our strong bond, we became two people searching for comfort and understanding, each projecting our own needs and fears onto this intentionally abstract piece of art.

The origins of Nicki's pain were no longer a mystery. Nicki had felt the signs before she and her father and the world could see and know the signs. Her school refusal reflected her internal mandate to stay by her mother's side. Like a gladiator, she tried to stave off the invasion. Like a child, she tried to soak in every moment she could with as much of her mother as she could hold onto.

And what of my contribution, my internal unrest? I believe it was twofold. First, like Nicki, I intensely experienced feelings of helplessness and frustration and shared her prison of knowing and not knowing at the same time. We watched separate yet not separate tragedies unfold, each feeling powerless to intervene and change the course of events. She watched her mother slip away despite Nicki's sacrifice and vigilant guarding. I watched Nicki slip away, to the prison of her home, to a therapeutic day program, then a residential school, and to what looked like a psychotic level of disorganization. As Nicki felt that she failed her mother, I felt that I had failed Nicki. I was unable to understand what Nicki could not articulate. I was unable to help her take up arms in her silent war.

Secondly, my feelings of vulnerability were triggered in my work with Nicki. My own fears of maternal loss stirred a kicking of anxiety in me that I struggled to keep out of the treatment room. I believe it was a blend of simmering raw anxiety and desperation, mine and hers, that propelled me out of my chair that morning and created our "moment of meeting" (Boston Change Process Study Group, 2010).

While magical, our "moment" did not single-handedly transform Nicki from a young woman incapacitated by anxiety and depression to a successful college student. Nicki's rich internal world had stayed strong, offering her comfort and the capacity to play during this terrible time. Her steady, supportive relationship with her father sustained and motivated her. Our relationship, my years of bearing witness to her confusion and pain, the gentle prying and prodding that I could rarely resist doing, and my willingness to join her in play kept Nicki connected to a me as a strong maternal figure and carrier of hope. I believe, however, that something in the moment Nicki and I shared, standing in front of that picture, brought her to the tipping point of change.

How do we understand the "forever," the years in which time seemed to stand still and Nicki showed little progress despite our work together? Perhaps it was a daughter's long goodbye to her beloved mother, her way of holding on even when nothing more than memories were left. In the stillness of this long regression, Nicki used play to build our relationship and slowly loosen the vise-like grip of her severe depression. Eventually, she became able to let her mother go, risking that I and others in her world would be there to make this terrifying aloneness bearable. It was in the "forever" of our work together that trust and understanding and love grew, and the relational magic was created. It was the "forever" that made the transformative power of the "moment" possible.

Today, I sit in session with Nicki, and she talks to me about which classes she will take next semester. Abnormal psychology, social psychology, child development. . . . all the classes that an aspiring child psychologist will need. I no longer am the impaired, helpless mother of those terrible years. Today, she experiences me in a new way, as someone with whom she can identify and in whose eyes she can see the pride and hope that fuel her surge forward.

For my part, there are moments when I fight to hold back my tears, experiencing a love and admiration for this young woman who has emerged so spectacularly from the swirl of a seven-year nightmare. She was her mother's fierce protector, her father's loyal companion, and my storyteller extraordinaire who stewarded us through the long storm. I struggle to feel pride in the work that I have done with Nicki, as holding on for dear life to simply stay connected was as much strategy as I could muster for much of our time together. But sometimes, I realize, just holding on can be everything. Just surviving the long stretches of wordless despair so that Nicki had a witness and companion in her misery allowed me to be a good enough therapist for Nicki. She held me in her mind through the fog of forever, when day and night were interchangeable, and reached for my hand when movement miraculously became possible.

For sure, Nicki still experiences much sadness and anxiety. She still avoids much of what smacks of separation. But time has picked up its fickle pace, and there is much movement. There is strength, there is humor, there is determination, and there is so much hope.

If I Could Turn Back Time

My work with Nicki supported my belief in the curative powers of the therapeutic relationship. It was my ability to "companion" (Grossmark, 2018) Nicki through her years of school refusal and the horrific two years of caring for her mother that helped her survive her mother's devastating decline and death. And it was my serving as a mother who was alive for Nicki, relishing her special gifts and offering patience, understanding, and determination, that proved instrumental to her survival and, eventually, to her surge toward health.

I felt Nicki's pain and the impossibility of the bind she found herself in. Yet I simply had no idea what was causing her pain or what opposing forces were paralyzing her. But Nicki was forgiving of my inability to understand what she was unable to put into words and my resulting misattunement. She expressed little disappointment or rancor at my inability to see what only she could see in the earliest phase of her mother's illness. Nicki didn't seem to feel judged or pressured by my weekly questions about her refusal to go to school, but neither did she make any attempt to answer them. It was as if, in her silent avoidance, she was patiently insisting, "You're asking the wrong questions. I need you to be smarter!"

If I could turn back time, I would indeed try to be smarter and more attuned to Nicki's experience. When I briefly chatted with her mother at the beginning of most sessions, she seemed worried and frustrated but cognitively intact. Looking back, however, I can remember attending a Committee on Special Education meeting for Nicki and noticing that when her mother paused to answer a question, Nicki jumped in and answered it for her. It was only a half-second pause, but this brief interaction registered with me. At the time, I assumed it reflected Nicki's impatience with her mother and with the very long meeting that was underway. In hindsight, I understand that Nicki's completing her mother's sentence and her determination to stay by her mother's side rather than attend school were her desperate attempts to protect her failing mother – in the only ways she could.

Thinking back, I wonder if my anxiety about my own mother's health interfered with my attunement to Nicki and her mother. I didn't notice the very subtle signs of Nicki's mother's decline, and I failed to question whether Nicki's desperate need was to be by her mother's side rather than to avoid school. Perhaps my terror at the idea of losing my own mother caused me to not see, not know, and not even consider the possibility that there might be something terribly wrong with Nicki's mom. My unconscious fear colluded with Nicki's unconscious mandate to protect her mother by keeping her decline a secret. Because this long *in*-actment was driven by the fear of losing a most precious and depended-upon source of love and support for both of us, it did not easily give way to conscious awareness, much less expression in words. This unconscious relational bind of not saying, not seeing, and not knowing was only loosened through action in a magical moment of aliveness between us.

If I could turn back time, I would understand my growing frustration and anger with Nicki's unremitting school refusal, in part, as a projective identification. I believe that Nicki's frustration and anger around finding herself in this bind – this need to take care of her mother at the expense of her own development – was too much for Nicki. She needed to induce these same feelings of helplessness and frustration in me, which I readily accepted given my own concerns about my mother. Had I understood this better at the time, I could have helped Nicki acknowledge and work through her feelings of fear, desperation, and anger at having to make this sacrifice and feeling like she had to do so in silence and isolation.

When Nicki began college and fully returned to the land of the living, I followed her in her rapid movement forward and tried to stay closely attuned to her anxiety, depression, and rapidly shifting sense of herself. My focus was on sharing with her my support and admiration as well as being a strong maternal and professional role model from whom she could learn – meeting her need for a mirroring and idealizable figure in her life. If I had it to do over again, I would explore Nicki's fears around issues of separation and autonomy more in the latter part of our work together. Though we discussed her avoidance of dating and learning to drive and paid attention to the role of her anxiety in both, we didn't speak about her fear of separation from her father and the internal mandate she now felt to stay by his side. Just as she had felt compelled to protect her mother through her long decline, she now felt the same need to sacrifice fully separating as a young adult so she could continue to emotionally protect her father.

I also chose not to explore our moment in front of the painting with Nicki. Months after this moment, I told myself that Nicki needed to fully own her miraculous turnaround rather than see it as a product of both her hard work and our connection. In truth, I think a part of me didn't want to shine the bright light of therapeutic inquiry on that moment for fear that to do so might rob it of its magic. What if Nicki experienced that moment and the moments that followed in the session differently than I did? What if she attributed her sudden turnaround to factors that I was unaware of? I think I simply didn't want to know. If I could turn back time, I would be braver and more confident in my experience of what transpired between us in the room that day. At the right time, I would share my experience in front of the painting with Nicki, and I would talk with her about the curative forces that I believe came from our strong, close bond.

References

The Boston Change Process Study Group. (2010). *Change in psychotherapy. A unifying paradigm*. W.W. Norton and Company.

Grossmark, R. (2018). *The unobtrusive analyst: Explorations in psychoanalytic companioning*. Routledge.

3   A Better Man

Introduction

It was a warm July afternoon, and I, my husband, and our two young children were enjoying ourselves on our small family boat. We were trying to anchor the boat when conflict erupted. When instructed to do so, I took out the boat's rear anchor, and with great effort, I heaved it into the water. I neglected, however, to secure the anchor to the anchor line, and as soon as the large metal structure left my hands, I realized that it would now be a permanent fixture on the floor of the Great South Bay of Long Island. My husband, stunned by my carelessness, began barking at me. Within seconds, my five-year-old son stood up between us. With his little hands on his hips, he turned to my husband and glared. Then, without missing a beat, he looked at me and demanded, "Marry someone else!"

Louis was disturbed by the burst of conflict, but he felt secure enough with his father to confront him – and to protect me. When he did so, he saw the gleam in his father's eyes responding to his little man's valor. Feelings of self-confidence rather than shame developed in Louis as a result of interactions such as this one.

In contrast, my patient Brian, a twenty-eight-year-old substance abuser, had a very different experience as a young boy. He was too traumatized as a child by his father's rage and brutality to raise his voice in protection of his battered mother. Crushing feelings of fear and shame derailed his emotional development, especially the development of his self-esteem. It was this shame that was buried deep beneath his self-hate and pummeling substance abuse.

Brian captured my attention from the moment he entered my office. With short red hair, deep blue eyes, and a muscular frame, he oozed a vitality that belied his long, damaging history of drug and alcohol addiction. I tried to help Brian understand that he was playing out his father's legacy of rage and violence and felt that he didn't deserve love or success. I raced to help him understand his unconscious mandate for self-destruction before he blew up the new life that he was struggling to build.

In the process, I colluded with Brian's wish for me to "not know," and together, we turned a blind eye to his dangerous downward spiral. This

DOI: 10.4324/9781003543343-4

chapter examines the interplay between my conscious and unconscious self-states and those of my patient and how the resulting enactments and *in*-actments both jeopardized and energized our work together.

A Better Man

I got the early-morning phone call two full years into my treatment with Brian and six short months after his wedding. Brian sounded desperate on the phone as he asked if I could have an emergency session with him and his wife. Later that afternoon, the couple sulked into my office and sat in silence. Brian's handsome, boyish face was cradled in his hands. Colleen looked fragile, perched tensely on the edge of her seat, her hands clasped tightly around a ball of tissues.

"Who would like to start?" I asked as I breathed in air thick with disappointment and despair.

After a long pause, Brian raised his tear-filled eyes to meet mine and began, "I'll start. I've been lying to both of you. Hell, I've been lying to myself. I've been using since before the wedding. Pills and coke mostly. I couldn't tell you why. I was happier than I've ever been in my life, but in the strangest fucking way, I felt like I was losing myself. I felt like I was becoming one of those guys we always made fun of growing up – the guy that wasn't mad all the time but the kind of guy we called a loser. But the truth is, I'm a fucking liar and a coward and a drug addict. She doesn't deserve the shit I put her through – none of it. I wanted to be different, but I'm just like my asshole father, and now, I'm gonna lose the most important person in the world to me. I'm so sorry. I hate myself for what I've done. That's all I have to say." With that, his head was once again in his hands, and I watched him take slow, deep breaths.

I let the silence fill the air. Brian had struggled in sessions with his sobriety and with once and for all stepping out of his father's shoes. I tried to quiet my own feelings of surprise, worry, and responsibility. But my thoughts persisted. How could I have missed this? Why had I naively believed Brian would be different from other substance abusers that I've treated? I shifted in my seat as I silently struggled with the prickly thorns of disappointment and self-reproach. *Not now,* I chided myself. *Right now, I need to stay in their world.*

As I looked over at Colleen, I saw her biting her lip in a struggle for composure. Her fair skin was blotchy from distress, and her light-blue eyes were puffy from crying. She was more petite than I had imagined, and I could see the softness and gentle beauty that Brian had described falling in love with. Finally, Colleen began, "This isn't the man that I married. This man broke my heart. Where did my Brian go? Where did the strong, protective, hard-working man that I fell in love with go? We've been married for six months, and it's been one lie after another. I'm working two jobs so he can stick that garbage up his nose. I'm really an idiot. I'm making him soup because I think he has the flu. I can't go through this anymore. It's all been a lie. I feel like the stupidest person on the planet." Colleen abruptly stopped talking and looked up at me for confirmation that I understood the depth of his betrayal and the rawness of her pain.

When our session together neared the end, I felt a need to offer her a modicum of hope and reassure her that it was not her job to put this man back together again. I also felt the urge to shake Brian and scream, "How could you do this? How could you ruin all OUR hard work?" I settled on telling them, "I'm so sorry that you two are going through this. Brian, my friend, you have a tremendous amount of work to do. We are going to have to double down on our work, and we need to talk about you going to twelve-step meetings."

"Absolutely," he immediately responded and then added, "Whether you throw me out on my ass or not, I swear to you I am done with this shit."

Colleen was silent as errant tears escaped her pale eyes and lined her delicate face.

"Colleen, I can see how horrible this has been for you. I know right about now, part of you is ready to kill him, at least ready to throw him out on his ass, as he put it. Is there a part of you that feels like you can give Brian some time to see if he can rediscover the man you fell in love with?" I asked.

Colleen was understandably unsure about her ability to forgive Brian but nodded in agreement. Seemingly with this simple gesture, the dam broke, and she began to sob.

As I sat in session, my heart ached for both of them, and I wondered whether their relationship could survive, even if Brian managed to stay sober. I questioned why, in the wake of learning about his relapse and ongoing deception, I felt sadness and guilt – but not the anger I would have expected. My thoughts went to the Brian I met two years ago and the stories that he told me. Before I continue with their story, let me tell you about Brian.

His mother's head made a sound somewhere between a crack and a thud as the rounded toe of his father's work boot repeatedly crashed into it. "She's okay, she's okay," ten-year-old Brian chanted softly to himself – half prayer, half glide into a familiar haze. As the beating continued, Brian's mind silently divided in two. He was dazzled by his crazy father, who often called him a junior version of himself. His mother, though, was his heart. She insisted on strict bedtimes and an endless list of chores for Brian, their only child. His mother cooked, cleaned their tiny home, and took care of Brian despite working twelve-hour shifts at a nearby diner.

Brian squeezed his eyes shut and stood frozen in place. Within moments, it was over, and the little boy was whisked back to the bar with his father and his father's friends. "Fucking bitch," his father wailed as he held court with the other unruly men, most clad in the outerwear of those who fixed or cleaned the spoils of others. "Stupid bitch won't bother me tonight," he added defiantly. Brian wanted to laugh with these brash, reckless men – to be one of them and share in their daily victories over the nagging women and demeaning bosses who held them down. At the same time, he wanted to stab his father's leg with the knife that sat by his plate of food, the leg that drove the boot that had savaged his mother's head just moments before. When his father pushed a beer in front of him, offering, "here, little man, show these fools how it's done," Brian's mind danced with glee, and like a child given cotton candy at Asbury Park, all felt right in his ten-year-old world.

Brian was raised in South Jersey in a small town near Cape May. He was the only child of his alcoholic father and his long-suffering mother. Brian's father, James, worked construction during the day and drank and sold drugs at night. His mother, Cheryl, was a waitress at a nearby diner and spent her time working long shifts and looking after Brian. Brian both admired and resented his mother's strength. Though she stood up to his father's drunken tirades, she never had the courage to leave him and was too proud to tell friends and relatives about the violence that was shattering their small world.

As James's drinking escalated, his violence toward Cheryl shifted from an insecure man's bullying to a predator's raw brutality. Little Brian felt a swirl of hatred, fear, and shame toward this larger-than-life creature that battered his mother's face and lunged in a drunken rage at his Little League coach when he benched Brian during a game. Despite this burden of shame and hate, Brian was also overwhelmed with feelings of specialness and excitement when he rode high on his father's shoulders and was introduced at the barber shop and the bars as "my little man."

Brian was an active and angry boy. His teachers and coaches admired his natural athleticism and bright mind but were unable to manage his unchecked energy and aggressive behavior. Brian was extremely sensitive to any slights and would bully boys who didn't readily defer to him. Deep down, he could feel what those who knew the family could see – the seeds of his father's rage and cruelty were beginning to take root inside of him.

Growing up, Brian was constantly stressed by the violence that filled his home. His salvation was a group of close friends, the neighborhood boys who ran wild through their small town. Brian and his friends were fiercely loyal to each other. He felt their caring when his friends generously ignored the humiliating public scenes that his drunken father would cause and took him into their homes when the fighting between his parents was particularly bad.

As a teenager, Brian felt the conflict between being the good boy that his mother was trying to raise and the feelings of power and excitement that his father's world seemed to promise. Time after time, Brian chose the illusion of strength and power over the whisperings of his conscience. His identification with his father, however, cost him dearly. By the end of high school, Brian was a raging bull who relied on drugs and drinking to manage his anger and firm up his fragile ego. Despite his bravado, Brian knew he was a fraud. Even as a teenager, he could feel his hunger for his father's approving glances. In his quietest moments, he had flickers of awareness of his self-hatred for not protecting his mother – and for having a close relationship with his father despite his abusiveness with his mother.

Brian graduated high school and went to a community college. As his drinking and drug use continued to escalate, he was quickly overwhelmed by the academic demands of school. Rather than face possibly failing his classes, Brian dropped out just before the Christmas break. With the distraction of school gone, Brian drank hard, smoked daily, and sold drugs to stay flush with cash and reassure himself that he was not the loser that much of the town thought he was.

Brian got a job with a construction crew during the day, and like his father, he gambled and dealt drugs out of two neighborhood clubs at night. He had short relationships with suffocating women and long relationships with unavailable ones. Brian was keenly aware of how busy he was going nowhere. A part of him was desperate for a chance to become a different kind of man. When he walked into my office, I sensed that Brian was searching for just that opportunity.

Brian was referred to me by his physician after calling him for sleeping pills. Realizing that there was more to his difficulties than trouble sleeping, his doctor suggested that Brian give me a call. At twenty-eight, Brian was a tall, muscular man of Irish descent, with short red hair and sharp blue eyes. He was strikingly handsome, made only more attractive by the vulnerability in his downcast stare when his thoughts strayed into the forbidden areas of his mind that were filled with shame and guilt.

Brian began our first session by focusing on his worsening feelings of anxiety and difficulty sleeping. He quickly pivoted, however, and voiced concern about his escalating use of cocaine and pills. As I listened to his stories of drug dealing, substance abuse, womanizing, and explosive rage, I wondered what change would look like for this man and how I was going to help him get there.

I liked Brian immediately. His quasi-criminal, bad-boy persona made his curious intellect and an unusual access to deep feelings a welcome surprise. A few weeks into our work, Brian began to share stories about his childhood and the horrors he witnessed with his abusive, alcoholic father. "Every holiday was a nightmare even though you hoped this time would be different. My mother would set up a Christmas tree, and I would help her decorate it. She would make a ham and a turkey and invite my grandparents and my aunt, uncle, and cousins over. Even though we didn't have a lot of money, she would buy presents for everyone. It would always start out okay. Then, every year, he would start drinking at lunch, and by dinner, he would be telling her that the food sucked and saying shit in front of her family to embarrass her. He would make a big deal over giving her some piece of jewelry, but he was such an asshole about it. He would practically throw it at her as he was saying shit. When she would get upset or just not make a fuss about it, he would throw a huge fit about how ungrateful she was. Then, like a fucking asshole, he would storm out and meet his loser friends at the bar. Merry fucking Christmas!"

Brian seemed to tell these stories to share the traumas of his childhood and explain why his perceived betrayal of his mother was unforgivable. "Why can't we leave him?" the frightened child in him longed to ask his mother. "How fucking stupid are you?" the rageful teenager in him wanted to scream at her. But he swallowed these words long before they formed in his mouth.

When Brian's father whisked him away for an afternoon, a weekend or, when he was older, weeks at a time, Brian's heart and mind would simply split in two.

"What was it like for you when you went off with your father?" I asked.

"What do you mean?" Brian shot back defensively. "It was crazy. He wasn't asking. I had to go with him when he told me to. Some days, I would watch he and his friends beat the shit out of a bunch of lowlifes from another town. Other times, we would hang in the bar with his friends and play darts all day. Sometimes, I wanted to go, but lots of times, I didn't. But it wasn't my choice."

After a long pause, I held his gaze and said, "I know it wasn't your choice, but do you?"

"I should have stood up for her," he snapped. "I should have told him to go fuck himself. I should have killed him a long time ago. I thought about it, lots of times. I pictured stabbing him with the knife that my mother used to carve ham. I could see myself slamming the blade into his chest, over and over. I could feel it crunch through his bones. I was just too much of a coward," Brian protested loudly.

After another long pause, I offered, "You have so much shame about not rescuing your mother; about loving your father."

"I should have protected her. I was a fucking coward," he insisted.

"No, Brian, you were a kid-in an impossible situation," I firmly told him.

Brian looked up at me, began to speak, and then stopped. He seemed to be trying to take in my words, and I saw him swallow hard.

As I struggled to help Brian develop empathy for the little boy and teenager he used to be, I was aware of my own strong feelings of protectiveness and caring for him. I felt the urge to hug Brian, a mother's hug to contain his pain and convince him of the good I saw inside of him. I surprisingly had little interest in exploring the explosive, self-sabotaging, or deceptive parts of Brian. It was as if by exploring Brian's more alarming and destructive self-states, I would lose sight of the little boy whose development had been hijacked by his father's brutality.

If I couldn't hold the different self-states of this man, how could I help him "stand in the spaces" between the competing versions of himself (Bromberg, 1998) and understand why he might sabotage his new life? How could I help him experience his extraordinary conflict between the powerful, drug-abusing, father self-state within him and the part of him that desperately wanted to be a good man, who could need and care in a loving relationship?

In hindsight, I believe Brian's relationship with his father triggered my own memories of growing up with my father. Unlike Brian's father, my father was a very good, loving man with a very quick temper. His anger was expressed verbally and was generally directed at me rather than my mother or siblings. I couldn't understand why my dangerous acting out and poor grades were ignored yet lights left on in the kitchen routinely provoked a harsh response. In the face of what seemed to my child self to be his frightening volatility and pointless criticism, I struggled to hold onto the loving sides of my father that he sometimes tried to share with me. It wasn't until I had my own children that I could embrace the devoted, playful, and adoring grandfather he had become.

As our work continued, Brian spoke about how he atoned for not defending his mother and for abandoning her to be with his father as an older adolescent. He proudly described spending the better part of his twenties visiting his mother on Wednesday nights for dinner, filling her small apartment with heartfelt gifts, and occasionally joining her for Sunday church. Brian felt he had finally become the good son he had always wanted to be, the son that his mother deserved. He would bring girlfriends over to meet her and talked about one day getting a house in which she would have her own apartment and help with the grandchildren. Brian couldn't imagine marrying any of these girls, but he saw the joy that these promises brought to his mother's eyes.

As an adult, Brian was disgusted by his father and repulsed by the similarities that he believed they still shared. Long gone were the feelings of excitement or specialness he used to feel by his father's side. Once he reached his mid-twenties, Brian had stopped speaking to his father and shuddered at the memory of how he used to admire him.

Toward the end of his first year in therapy, Brian's mother died tragically from a sudden heart attack. The two shared a close relationship in her final years, and Brian took comfort knowing that he had become an involved, supportive part of her life. While Brian spent many sessions mourning his mother's loss and talking about the guilt that still burdened him, he was finally starting to question the old, bone-deep feelings of self-hatred he felt for not protecting his mother. Perhaps it was his father who deserved his rage and not himself, we considered together. Just maybe, he had done the best he could at the time.

As Brian began to forgive himself for the sins of his father and his inability to protect his mother, he began to consider that he might deserve what he called "a good life." In our sessions, he started focusing more intensively on his drug use. He was disgusted with himself for his cocaine and pill use but was clear that he wasn't ready to stop drinking or smoking pot. These were the childhood friends that he relied on for comfort when he was flooded with feelings of anger or regret. Sometimes, he shared, he felt like weed and whiskey were the only things that prevented him from killing someone, anyone, just to quiet the storm that raged inside him.

"It's the fucking coke and pills I can't say no to. It happens so quickly. This guy on one of the other crews comes up when we're on break and presses two Vicodins in my hand. 'Long fucking day,' he says. 'No, man, I'm good,' I say. 'I know you are, you're the man,' he answers, and he winks and walks away. Next day, I'm buying another bottle from him. I tell him I'm cutting this shit out soon, that I'm gonna get 'healthy,' but we both know I'm full of shit."

"Are you full of shit, or are there just different Brians inside you, one that wants to burn everything down and one that very much wants to get his life together?" I asked.

"Maybe," he said, "but the first guy is winning, and I feel like time is running out."

"Go on," I prodded.

With that, Brian talked softly, almost sadly, about the wonderful girl he was dating, the promotion he was eying at work, and the conversations that he had with the mother who lives on in his mind.

"Those are real too, as real as the Vicodin," I offered. "Tell me more about Colleen."

Perhaps it was the vulnerability he was feeling with me after talking about his disappointment in himself, perhaps it was his fear of the real closeness that he was heading toward with Colleen, but a different Brian showed up for the following session. Brian walked into my office about ten minutes late with red eyes and a defiant stare. "Hey, Doc," he smirked, "S'happening? Sorry – running a little late."

"What should I make of that? You're never late," I asked and then added, "And you never came to a session stoned before."

"Nah, I'm not stoned. I just had a long fucking day. You got me all wrong this time," Brian assured me.

"Really?" I asked incredulously. "You're going to try to play me now? So much easier than feeling vulnerable with me."

"Fuck you!" he snapped. "I don't need your shit. I don't need this shit at all."

I met Brian's challenge and responded, "I think 'this shit' is exactly what you need, just not when you're stoned. So why did you come fucked up to our session?"

After an unusually long silence, which I was determined not to break, Brian answered, "It's just easier to do what I've always done. It's just who I am."

After another long minute, I quietly said, "It's only one part of you. But I think you wanted to make sure we both knew that side of you is still alive and kicking."

I understood that Brian's drug use soothed his deep shame and volcanic rage. It was also an important self-state within him that felt like a central part of his identity. I believed that his ongoing use also protected him from his fear of depending on anyone and from his dangerously low self-esteem. And I knew if he continued to use pot and alcohol as his mainstay for coping, he would never learn more adaptive ways of managing his explosive emotional life.

Over the next year, Brian used our work together, episodic twelve-step meetings, and much determination to stop using hard drugs, get a promotion at work, and cut down substantially on his drinking. Rather than pressing him to give up all substances, I relaxed my usual focus on abstinence and appreciated the herculean push toward health that Brian was making. By focusing on his capacity to change, I hoped to strengthen his sense of agency and his self-esteem. Perhaps part of me also feared his anger as well as my concern about being experienced as another critical figure in his life.

Toward the end of this very productive second year of therapy, Brian announced that he was on the precipice of something truly terrifying: he and Colleen were engaged. Over the year they'd been dating, Brian described her as having a softness and kindness that made his heart melt. I learned that Colleen was a second-grade teacher who had never been married, and the two dreamed of having a home and a family together. This idea both thrilled and terrified Brian, as he was painfully aware of his potential to repeat his father's mistakes.

Brian described talking for hours with Colleen and sharing with her the awful details of how he grew up. He spoke about his fear that deep inside, he was rotten like his father. What he didn't share was that he worried about his habit of sleeping with other women, particularly when he was drinking.

"Kind of playing Russian roulette with Colleen's heart and your own," I observed.

"I know," he said. "It would kill me to hurt her. Girls have always been so available for me. I know I'm an asshole like that. I don't ever want to hurt her."

I wondered with Brian whether this was his emotional exit ramp, one more way he reassured himself he could still be the fuck-up his father had raised him to be.

Once the couple became engaged, Brian committed to being "almost clean." For him, this meant that he smoked pot when he had trouble sleeping but no longer drank or used hard drugs. With this change, he explained, he also wouldn't be tempted to be with other women, something he was determined not to do again. I felt encouraged by Brian's commitment to leave alcohol and more toxic drugs behind and embrace his new life with his Colleen and their Border Collie puppy, Oscar.

As the months went on, however, Brian began to describe periodic fights in which he would explode, Colleen would cry, and he would feel "like the worst piece of shit in the world." These fights eventually resolved with his tearful apologies, and the couple continued their march toward marriage. Brian's dreams, no longer sandcastles, were finally being built on firm ground.

Blinded by my hope for his future and my feelings of pride for the hard work we'd done together, I was unable to see that Brian was beginning the process of blowing up his new life.

The months leading up to the wedding fast became weeks and then days. Our sessions were filled with hope as Brian described a connection with Colleen and an experience of happiness that he had never thought possible. We talked at length about how his father was still lurking in the shadows within him and his own process of self-forgiveness that was palpably incomplete. We anticipated triggers for his hot temper and the irresistible pull of self-sabotage, be it with drugs, alcohol, other women, or his own temper.

While the wedding was everything that Colleen and Brian had hoped for, their first six months of marriage were very rough. The couple began to have frequent arguments. Colleen would question Brian's moodiness, and he would scream and punch walls. These arguments were followed by deadly silences that often lasted days.

Six months after their wedding, Brian missed work for three days in a row. He was still sleeping each morning when Colleen was ready to leave for school. The second morning, she gently woke him to see how he was feeling. "Get the fuck off of me," he barked at her and rolled over, pulling his pillow over his head. Like the day before, Brian disappeared until late in the evening and didn't respond to Colleen's calls or texts. She waited up for him on the third night and confronted him. Angry and frightened, Colleen cried, "What is the matter with you? Where are you going every night? I don't like this Brian. This isn't what I signed up for. Please, tell me what's going on with you?"

"Now you're my fucking mother? I didn't sign up for a warden. How about cutting me a break and leaving me the fuck alone," an angry Brian bellowed.

A week later, Brian's coke dealer came to their house looking for the ten thousand dollars Brian owed him, and Colleen began to put the pieces together. Three days later, the couple walked into my office, and together, we stumbled through the wreckage of their young marriage.

Brian and I were in session the week following our joint meeting with Colleen, and he gave me the gory details of his recent drug use, chronic lying, and financial devastation. He ended with, "She hates me. She really hates me, and I deserve it. Now you fucking hate me too."

After a long pause, I looked at him and said, "Holy shit! I have a lot of different feelings right now – sadness, worry, frustration, but not hate. My guess is that you're the only one who hates you right now." After another minute of silence, I asked, "How do you understand what you've been doing?"

Brian told me the story of his spiral out of control, which started just weeks after the wedding. The couple decided against a honeymoon and put their money into buying a small house. "I felt like I was wearing someone else's shoes, living someone else's life. A wife, a yard, a dog. Really nice Italian leather, and they fit beautifully, but they weren't my shoes. I felt like a phony. When I started with a few Vicodin, I felt like I was myself again, and from there, it went to coke – lots and lots of coke. It was like nothing had changed at all; I felt like I was back in my own skin being the piece of shit I was meant to be." Brian explained.

"Who decides who or what you are meant to be?" I asked and after a brief pause added, "You or your father?"

Brian insisted on detoxing on his own. He welcomed the physical pain of withdrawal and managed the cravings that came fast and furiously. He felt the burn of Colleen's quiet anger and disappointment and the crushing weight of his own shame. Both the physical and the emotional pain of detox soothed his aching need to punish himself, and his ability to withstand the pain offered him a morsel of redemption. Colleen was neither throwing him out nor promising to work through this with him. She simply cried over the lies and the wasted thousands of dollars that forced her to take on a second job.

Suddenly aware of the *in*-actment that Brian and I had been engaged in, I thought long and hard about the parent/child dance we had learned to do so well. His longing to make me proud and fear of disappointing me led to his silence about his escalating drug use. My approving gaze felt healing to him, as if my admiring view was proof of his goodness. For my part, I so wanted Brian to have the life he finally dared to dream of, and I wanted to feel that I helped him achieve this. I realized that I had stopped searching for clues that he was using drugs again and no longer listened closely for what wasn't being said. Absent still were my negative feelings – my anger at being lied to or my shame at being fooled. I had to ask both Brian and myself why we had colluded to keep his devastating downfall outside of our awareness in the treatment room.

Brian talked about how badly he wanted me to see him as a changed man and how desperately he wanted to be that changed man. I spoke again with him about my sense that there were different Brians within him: the man in my office who fought through his deep pain and was committed to sobriety and the man who lied to anyone who cared about him and leaned hard on drugs and alcohol to survive in his tumultuous emotional world – to name a few. I owned my shame for being asleep at the wheel and not seeing his downfall as it happened. I guessed that it was my wanting so much more for him and my belief in him, both of which still stood strong, that closed my eyes to the subtle signs. I also wondered aloud if we were both afraid that his father's shadow and his longstanding reliance on drugs were too crippling for us to manage.

Together, we agreed to pivot in our work together. I would ask him details about his recovery each week and voice even my slimmest concerns. I wouldn't give up on him if he continued to use, and I wouldn't be swayed by his anger. For his part, he needed to bring all his feelings, including his anger, into our sessions. Things might get ugly, I warned both of us, but we would survive it together.

Brian was able to stay sober but was losing patience with Colleen's constant suspicion and coldness. He took on a second job to stay busy and avoid her diminishing gaze. The couple no longer fought often, but there was little laughter and even less sex. After six months of sobriety, Brian felt that his emotional debt had been paid, and righteous indignation filled the treatment room. The lack of warmth and conversation between them made Brian feel that Colleen would always hate him. The lack of sex made him feel like less of a man, like there was nothing he had to offer that she still wanted.

In one session, Brian had clenched his fists and spat as he shouted at me, "I'm fucking sick of it. She just keeps bringing up the past, over and over and over. I'm not that guy anymore, but she just keeps acting like I'm a piece of shit. If I sleep in once a month, she thinks I'm getting high again," Brian wailed.

"Why on earth would she think that?" I wondered aloud, thinking about how his drug use had savaged their relationship.

Brian calmed slightly with my familiar sarcasm. "Fuck her," he said, this time with the sadness of a defeated man. "She's never gonna trust me. She's never gonna want me again."

"Remind me," I asked, "How long were you an asshole?"

Brian looked up at me and said with a childlike lilt in his voice, "A few years, I guess. Pretty much the whole time I've known her."

Matching his soft tone, I countered, "Right now, she's too afraid to hope. Just like you are."

Today, Brian is almost two years sober. He is still working hard in therapy, trying to understand and manage his lifelong feelings of anger, guilt, and shame. Brian and Colleen are struggling to find their way back to each other, and both seem committed to saving their marriage. He continues to battle his volatile temper and pushes himself to talk about his feelings before he is shouting or punching walls. Colleen is working on forgiving her husband and letting herself see, with fresh eyes, the man that he is fighting to become. They have taken up jogging together and, at least monthly, they go together to Sunday church. Despite all the pain and conflict, Brian is determined to be the man his mother and wife believed he could be – the man I hoped he could be. Brian is bone tired from struggling on so many fronts. But for now, he sleeps the uninterrupted sleep of a better man.

If I Could Turn Back Time

Brian's volatility and reliance on substances to manage painful affect made looking into his emotional world a risky endeavor. It was unclear whether Brian would be able to tolerate the intimacy of therapy or the strong feelings that our work would inevitably trigger. Despite my concerns, we were able to develop a strong bond and navigate treacherous waters together. I was able to help Brian free himself from the shackles of his toxic identification with his father, his self-destructive use of drugs, and his shame-based volatility.

While Brian was able to use therapy to change the course of his life, there is still much to be learned by looking at what I could have done differently. If I could turn back time, I would catch myself sooner in our *in*-acted dance and recognize more quickly the unconscious forces behind my own need to "not know" when Brian was using again. By recognizing the self-hating side of him lurking in the shadows of his surge forward, I could have stemmed the tide of Brian's self-destructive acting out sooner. Had my feelings of competence and self-worth as a clinician not been so tied to Brian's climb toward emotional health and sobriety, I might have allowed myself to see the hidden signs of his resumed drug use much earlier.

My deep affection for Brian intensified my experience of "rooting for him" and my inclination to dive into the role of the admiring and encouraging therapist when he began to make important changes in his life. As our work progressed, I was determined to shore up his deficient self-esteem and focused on the "Brian in recovery" version of him that walked into my office each session. In doing so, I turned a blind eye to any signs of the addict side of him and stopped looking for the emotional unrest and destabilizing conflicts that were triggering his drug-abusing self-state.

Focusing exclusively on the patient's self-state that is succeeding in recovery is a common trap in substance abuse work and one that I fell into despite knowing better. I think my surprise and appreciation for how hard Brian was working to understand himself and free himself from the chains of addiction contributed to my relaxing my usual skepticism and vigilance with substance abuse patients. In hindsight, I would spend more time exploring how he was handling the stressors in his life, challenging his stubbornly negative self-image, and consistently checking in on his long-standing tendency to turn to drugs rather than people for the emotional relief he needed.

If I could turn back time, I would recognize my own anxiety about Brian's volcanic anger as well as my fear that he would abandon treatment if he experienced a rupture between us that triggered his intense feelings of shame. I would talk with Brian about this latter concern and would more directly invite the raging side of him into the treatment room (Davies, 1996, 1997, 1998). In doing so, I would hope to gain more direct access to the overwhelming feelings of helplessness that were underneath his shame and chronic drug use (Dodes, 2002). My ability to withstand his fury and my faith in our joint ability to repair our relationship would enable Brian to experience his anger as less deadly. And by experiencing my empathy and acceptance of this hated father part of himself, Brian could begin to integrate the very disparate parts of himself that had been splintered by early trauma.

Finally, if I could turn back time, I would focus more on Brian's emotional struggle as a victim of chronic childhood trauma. While he was quick to marinate in his anger toward his father and shame for not protecting his mother, Brian was unable to think or talk about his resentful or disappointed feelings toward his mother. I would help him become aware of his dissociated ire toward his mother for prioritizing her masochistic relationship with her husband over her need to protect her son. I believe this buried anger ate away at him, fueling his need for the relief that drugs offered and hindering his ability to have an intimate, mutual relationship with a woman. Similarly, his disappointment in his mother's inability to prioritize him and to protect him from his father's toxic influence made trusting others, including me, feel like a fool's pursuit.

References

Bromberg, P. (1998). *Standing in the spaces: Essays on clinical process, trauma, and dissociation*. The Analytic Press.

Davies, J.M. (1996). Linking the "pre-analytic" with the postclassical: Integration, dissociation and the multiplicity of unconscious process. *Contemporary Psychoanalysis*, 32: 553–576.

Davies, J.M. (1997). Dissociation, therapeutic enactment, and transference-countertransference processes: A discussion of papers of childhood sexual abuse by Sarnat and Grand. Pre-publication manuscript. *Gender and Psychoanalysis*, 2: 241–257.

Davies, J.M. (1998). Multiple perspectives on multiplicity. *Psychoanalytic Dialogues*, 8: 195–206.

Dodes, L. (2002). *The heart of addiction: A new approach to understanding and managing alcoholism and other addictive behaviors*. HarperCollins.

4 Chicken Parm

Introduction

My husband and I dated for what felt like an eternity before he finally proposed. It was 3:00 o'clock on a Saturday afternoon, halftime during a Boston College football game, and four years into our relationship when Jack brought a single red rose into the living room. He sat next to me on his old vinyl couch and asked me to share my life with him. "Yes!" I shrieked. "Yes!" I was ecstatic, and though I had known that this moment was coming, I was still oddly surprised.

Jack suggested we go to my favorite Boston restaurant, The Colorado Public Library, to celebrate. Several hours later, I was sipping a glass of cabernet, sharing an appetizer of fried calamari, and eagerly anticipating my blackened swordfish. He was asking if I wanted to go to his parents' house after dinner to share the good news when I noticed that my heart was beating uncomfortably fast. Within seconds, I started to feel queasy and headed for the bathroom. I hunkered down by the sink for at least twenty minutes with a cold compress on my head. I was doing my best to slow my racing heartbeat and ignore my nauseous stomach. I didn't think I was having a heart attack, but I was terrified by whatever was happening to me.

I finally made my way back to the table, looked at my now fiancé and the cold piece of swordfish in front of me, and ran back to the safety of the bathroom. This was my first panic attack, but it would not be my last. Certain developmental crossroads in my life, wonderful as the anticipated changes promised to be, caused tidal waves of anxiety that stopped me in my tracks. I have since learned to rely on daily exercise, my many dogs, and therapy to develop the insight and tools to fight back.

The next story, "Chicken Parm," details Daphne and Evan's struggle to take on the challenges of adulthood, including separation, individuation, and intimacy. Powerful symptoms of anxiety and feelings of demoralization were raging at this crossroads in their lives. These struggles chipped away at the core of their young marriage and brought them to my office.

This story also illustrates some of the difficulties a couple therapist faces when they find themselves empathizing more with one partner. In fact, it's

DOI: 10.4324/9781003543343-5

very common for a therapist to resonate more with one member of the couple's experience, especially when the conflicts at play trigger painful memories from the therapist's own past. Recognizing these feelings and the ruptures and enactments they may spark is crucial for the treatment to be successful.

Chicken Parm

Some couples come to marital therapy too late, after too much trust has been lost and far too much emotional damage has been inflicted. Almost no one comes too early. When a couple enters treatment with complaints that sound benign, it's time to start looking hard at what's lurking beneath the surface. Daphne and Evan had been married for four years when they walked into my office, but they had been together since the middle of high school, a full thirteen years ago. At twenty-nine, familiarity was breeding contentment for both of them – no passion, no excitement, but nothing too ugly either. Or so I thought.

Daphne began the first session in what I would learn was her typically overwhelmed and overwhelming manner. "Evan doesn't see me. He looks at me like I'm a piece of furniture, like I'm a piece of wood. He has nothing to say for himself either. He was always quiet, but now, he's practically mute. And he never wants to do anything except watch TV or lift his stupid weights," Daphne complained, as she gave Evan a look halfway between imploring and eviscerating.

After a long pause, I asked, "So you're feeling ignored, maybe unimportant?"

Daphne jumped on my words, "Like a piece of furniture. How important is that? I might as well just go to my parents'. At least they notice I'm there."

I let the silence fill the air and looked over at Evan, who had, in fact, been sitting practically mute since the beginning of the session.

Evan took my stare as a cue and quietly said, "You are always holding court with one problem or another, one thing after another that I didn't do right. It's exhausting. I gave up on normal conversation."

"That's the most he's said all month!" Daphne provocatively informed me, and then she gave a full-throttle description of the stressors connected to her high-powered job, her preoccupation with her health, and her need to "have things done a certain way!" "It's been awful," she continued. "I've always been a kind of high-strung, anxious person. It was bad before we got married, but the past year, my anxiety has gotten worse. We want to get pregnant, and we've been trying, but it doesn't help when I'm having a racing heartbeat and pains in my chest and he's looking at me like I'm a coffee table."

Daphne's anxiety and domineering manner already seemed to be taking over the session, and I was feeling like I had to fight for control in the room. She seemed desperate to feel heard and understood, and though I feared triggering another lengthy monologue, I said, "Tell me about your panic attacks."

"Sometimes, I wake up in the middle of the night and my heart is racing. It feels like it's going a million miles a minute. Other times, my chest feels tight, and sometimes, I even get chest pains. My mind starts racing, and it's terrifying. It doesn't happen when I'm at work, just at night when I'm trying to fall asleep. I went on Zoloft shortly before we got married because the panic attacks were getting so bad. It helped, but they're still happening," Daphne informed me.

"Tell her what you do when you wake up in the middle of the night," Evan prompted.

Daphne continued, "Sometimes, I wake Evan up to sit with me. They are really awful, and I get scared. He's my husband, for fuck's sake. I should be able to count on him. Lately, I was afraid that I was having a heart attack because of the pain, so he took me to the emergency room. Most of the time, he just sits with me and tells me stupid jokes. Big fucking deal."

"It is a big fucking deal. This shit happens three or four times a week, and we wind up in the ER a few times a month. I need to be on my game during the day, and it's exhausting. I don't complain, I'm just not conversation central," Evan defensively swung back.

"It sounds awful for both of you. I'm starting to get the picture of where things stand today. Let's get a little history. Can you tell me the story of your relationship?" I asked.

Not surprisingly, Daphne launched into her high-octane version of their story together. "We were in the same homeroom in eleventh grade, and it all started then. I kissed Evan at my best friend Barbara's party, and he asked me to be his girlfriend. He wasn't super popular or on any of the sports teams. He was cute, though, tall with those big blue eyes and I couldn't bear to hurt his feelings. We dated through the last two years of high school. Instead of being on a sports team like other guys, he worked a million hours a week at a gas station and always smelled a little like gasoline. It was embarrassing, but I put up with it. I broke up with him twice; once when this super-hot, super-popular senior asked me out when I was in eleventh grade, and I thought maybe I would get to go to the prom. The other time was when he wanted to go to college in Florida, and I thought it was an incredibly selfish decision. I knew that I wasn't going away to school, and I assumed that if Evan loved me, he would stay home too," Daphne stated, as if that was an obvious conclusion.

After barely taking a breath, she continued, "I went to NYU and lived at home, and Evan wound up going to Farmingdale State. I think I knew that we would get married since the beginning of college. My parents love Evan, but my mom always thought that I should have dated other guys before settling down. She was concerned about Evan's lack of ambition, and neither of us were so sure that he would ever make enough money. That's another issue we have – I'm the one who makes more of the money. Evan is always worried about money but not so much that he tries to make more of it."

Finally, and thankfully, Daphne took a breath, and I took the opportunity to check in with Evan. I was fast getting an impression that this five-foot, one-hundred-pound woman with piercing green eyes was an emotional pit bull, and I wondered if Evan was a little bit afraid of her. I know I was. "How do you feel about Daphne's description?" I asked Evan.

"We have been together forever. She's been my best friend forever. Yeah, all the details are right, but she makes it sound so basic. I gave up going to school in Tampa to go to school in Farmingdale. That was huge for me. It was my dream to go to school in Florida. I gave it up just so I could stay with Daphne. I couldn't believe that she wouldn't move in with me throughout college. She wouldn't even stay overnight in my apartment for years because Mommy and Daddy might get mad. But I dealt with it. I feel like I put up with a lot. Her breaking up with me because some dumb jock was into her for a hot second, at least that was over quickly. Daphne's anxiety and her constant criticism are the gifts that keep on giving," Evan quietly said.

Game on, I thought. Daphne and Evan were an interesting couple. I had the feeling that they had grown out of their high school and then college relationship, and neither seemed to have the slightest idea how to have an intimate adult relationship. They had been together for almost half of their twenty-nine years, and it seemed unimaginable to both that they wouldn't stay together. Perhaps, I thought, they have grown too comfortable with one another, and no one was bringing their A game to the relationship. Had she reverted to being the demanding, high-maintenance child she was with her father? Had he once again become the sulky, uncommunicative adolescent who was routinely nagged by his frustrated mother? These questions came to mind as I realized that I was feeling more like a parent in the room, trying to broker a truce between my two warring children.

Daphne was a petite, thin, very attractive young woman with shoulder-length blond hair that always looked like she'd just had a blowout. I learned that she came from a wealthy Jewish family from the North Shore of Long Island. Her mother worked part-time as a realtor, and she and Daphne had a close but slightly combative relationship. Her father was an orthopedic surgeon who clearly favored Daphne over her older sister, Debra. Daphne was a self-admitted Daddy's girl and was not used to asking twice for anything that she wanted, until that is, she married her middle-class, budget-conscious husband. Daphne graduated from NYU with a degree in marketing and worked long days in the PR department of a large law firm in the city. She thrived in the fast-paced, pressured environment of the law firm and was resolute that she would continue to work after she and Evan had a baby.

Evan was a pleasant-looking young man, with blue eyes, dark-blond hair, and dimples when he smiled. He was six feet tall, muscular, and the oldest of three boys. Evan graduated college and decided against pursuing graduate school in physical therapy as Daphne and her parents would have liked. He made a living as a personal trainer at a high-end gym and hoped to have private clients in the near future.

Evan grew up on the other side of town from Daphne, in a middle-class Irish Catholic family. He described having a conflictual relationship with his hard-to-please and very opinionated mother. He and his father were very close. Evan spoke admiringly about the older man's work ethic as the manager of a large supermarket and his patience with Evan's very critical mother. Like his father, Evan was a quiet guy who used TV, working out, and video games to manage his emotional world.

During our second session, I asked, "Tell me about your sex life together."

Not surprisingly, Daphne started, "Our sex life is okay. Not like in *Cosmo* but okay. Kind of like going to your neighborhood Italian restaurant and ordering chicken parm. You're never disappointed, but you're never surprised either. Lately, though, I haven't felt like chicken parm, and Evan hasn't even wanted to go to a restaurant."

"Chicken parm?" I repeated and then looked at Evan, who seemed to require an invitation to speak.

"So I'm a chicken parm? That's not terrible. I like chicken parm. Whatever. Our sex life is fine. Daphne wants sex all the time, but I keep telling her that I'm not a machine. Sometimes, I'm not in the mood or I'm exhausted. And when we have sex, it's always on Daphne's terms. It's always at night, always the same routine, and always the same position. I asked Daphne to try some new things, and she told me I'm ridiculous. This is Daphne's world. I'm just living in it," he responded in a resigned manner.

Both members of this couple felt much younger to me than their twenty-nine years. It seemed to me that the root of their problems came from a much earlier time and that issues from their own childhoods were still very much alive. I wanted to help Daphne understand the formidable anxiety that she struggled with. I suspected that her anxiety was connected to separating from her parents and her feelings of vulnerability and inadequacy in the face of adult pressures and developmental challenges. I hoped to get Evan to talk about his anger and how it was handled in his family growing up. I thought this was an emotion that both he and his father swallowed so often that it inhibited any passion or ambition. Without half of his emotional register, Evan's drive was in park, and he seemed to only be going through the motions in most aspects of his life.

I noted the long list of things I felt pressured to address with this couple as well as the uncharacteristic urge I felt to make a checklist. Like Evan, I realized that I was anxious about Daphne's impending criticism and was reacting like an insecure child scrambling to avoid their parent's admonishment. It felt too early in our work to share this with Daphne, as I feared it would replicate the kind of misattunement that she experienced with her husband.

As our sessions continued over the next few months, the couple sparred over Daphne's frequent disappointment in Evan's inability to provide sufficient emotional support and his lack of success as a provider. He wasn't enough – he didn't do enough, he didn't make enough, he didn't care enough, etc. I was cringing as Daphne pummeled her husband's self-esteem and couldn't stop myself from asking, "Daphne, what do you imagine it's like for Evan to hear about all the ways you feel he's failing you?"

"I can't imagine it matters very much to him. Otherwise, he might try a little harder to give me what I need," she angrily responded.

Determined to crack the shell of Daphne's self-absorption, I plodded forward. "Evan, can you tell your wife what it's like for you?"

Evan knew what I did not – that Daphne couldn't hear his answer to this question. Despite this, he took a few deep breaths before finally saying, "I just give up. It feels like I've loved Daphne my whole life. She knew I wasn't the smartest or funniest guy in the world. And she knew I wasn't going to be the richest. She was always going to make more money than me. I can't keep apologizing for that. Sometimes, I just give up and shut up."

Rather than reflecting on Evan's feelings, Daphne dug into her position as the victim and cited yet another example of how her husband had recently failed her. She vividly described the panic attack she'd had in the middle of the night two nights before. With loud, pressured speech, she explained that she woke with a jolt at three a.m., feeling like her heart was pounding out of her chest and she couldn't catch her breath. The familiar idea that she was having a heart attack suddenly consumed her thoughts, and her mind was racing with fears of her imminent death. She woke Evan up, crying that this time she was sure that she was having a heart attack, and they needed to go to the emergency room. Evan groggily pointed out that she was in the ER three nights prior, for the second time that month, and she was examined and was told she was having a panic attack. He told her to go back to sleep.

With uncharacteristic animation, Evan interrupted, "What she doesn't tell you is that I offered to stay up with her until she fell back to sleep, and she called me a lazy sack of shit who couldn't support a doorknob. Very nice!"

Daphne glared at both of us and, in doing so, confirmed my belief that she was preoccupied with trying to manage her own anxiety and was unable to feel any empathy for Evan's experience. She desperately needed to feel taken care of and still longed to be coddled, as she had been by her parents. As a result, she was easily overwhelmed and couldn't recognize Evan's attempts at being a supportive, caring partner.

I realized that I was having trouble summoning up the necessary empathy for Daphne. I made sure to validate how overwhelming the panic attacks were for her, but, truth be told, I almost had to force myself to do so. I knew I was having trouble feeling my way past Daphne's barbed-wire defenses and was emotionally much more aligned with Evan. Trying to recenter myself and gain greater access to Daphne's experience, I continued, "Wow. The whole situation sounds horrible for both of you. Your panic attacks seem to be the kind that really feel like a heart attack, regardless of what the ER doctor said. Thinking back on it now, what kind of response do you think you were hoping for from Evan?"

"I don't know. I guess telling me that he would stay up with me until I fell back to sleep was good, but it wasn't enough. He should have held my hand and reassured me that I was going to be okay, and we could go to the hospital in the morning if I still felt this way. I wanted him to take charge and make me feel taken care of – that's what would have helped," Daphne offered with a softer voice that made her sound like a frightened nine-year-old.

As Daphne's vulnerability came to the forefront, the grip that our enactment had on me began to loosen. I realized that I was not less immersed in Daphne's inner world, I was refusing to imagine Daphne's inner world at all. I was reacting to my experience of their interactions and was repelled by her self-absorption and harshness, much as Evan had been. As a result, I ignored her fragility, and like Evan, I too was rejecting Daphne's pleas for understanding and empathy.

Trying to repair the growing rupture between us (and model for Evan), I said to Daphne, "I think I've been missing the boat a bit. I got distracted by your anger at Evan, and that's not fair to you. Can you talk more about how Evan's responses have made you feel?"

"I felt like a I was an annoying child. I was being a pain yet again, and he was annoyed and wanted me to shut up and go back to sleep. He wasn't taking anything I said seriously."

"Kind of like you couldn't count on him – that you were too needy and you were on your own?" I asked.

"Exactly!" Daphne said, springing to life. "My parents never made me feel that way."

Again unexpectedly, Evan chimed in, "And there we have it, folks: one more way I don't live up to Papa James."

I felt the thunder of another impending storm and tried to stave it off. "Evan, I know feeling like you don't measure up to her father is a trigger for you, but can you stay with what Daphne is telling you she needs from *you*?" I asked – emphasizing the word "you."

With my question, Evan blinked and shifted uncomfortably in his seat. What followed was not his trademark passive silence. It was Evan's silent struggle to consider the possibility that maybe he could be enough and that both Daphne and I believed that he was capable of providing the emotional support that she needed.

We spent several sessions working on how each member of the couple understood and communicated what they needed from each other. I was feeling very positively about the progress that both Daphne and Evan were making in our work together when I got the weekend phone call.

"Dr. Feldman," Daphne barked into the phone, "that motherfucker has really done it now. He's a lowlife scumbag and a fucking loser, and I'm done with him." As Daphne continued her rant, I learned that Evan had been fired from his position as a personal trainer at a nearby, high-end gym when it came to light that he had been sexting with a seventeen-year-old-member whom he was training. Apparently, Daphne's friend was a member of the gym and was quick to deliver the locker-room gossip about her husband's "fucking around," the "dick pics," and how the girl's parents stormed the gym to complain to management about the pictures and texts they found on their daughter's phone. The combination of humiliation and feelings of betrayal were understandably overwhelming for Daphne, and this only exacerbated her underlying belief that she could only count on her father to take care of her.

My first thought upon hearing this news was that I now knew what Evan did with his anger. My second thought was, *oh shit!*

Daphne was understandably devastated and confronted Evan, demanding that he move out. Evan was tearful and extremely remorseful but insisted that he loved Daphne and would never have taken the flirting any further. He agreed to sleep in the guest room but was resolute that he would make this up to Daphne, and their marriage was not over. It became clear to me that Evan was not passive at all, and I had mistakenly bought the long-suffering, good-guy presentation that he offered. His sexting with his young client was one big "fuck you" to Daphne and a sign that he was drowning in feelings of anger and inadequacy – feelings that may have started in his childhood but were being triggered every day in his marriage.

Over the next month, I had individual sessions with both Daphne and Evan to try to keep this young marriage from falling apart. In our individual sessions, Evan talked about having to cater to Daphne's whims, whether it was her panic attacks, her shopping sprees, or her refusal to do any of the things that he liked to do. The sexting wasn't about sex, according to Evan; it was about having fun on his terms and someone finding him more exciting than "a piece of chicken parm."

As he talked about how sorry he was that he hurt his wife, I said, "But . . ."

Evan looked down and swallowed hard before he continued, "but she treats me like she treated me in high school. Like the kid who isn't good enough for her or her fucking family – like the kid who smells like the gas station – I'm tired of feeling like I don't measure up and she'll never see it."

"This is the anger that's been missing from our sessions," I said. "I only hear about Daphne's anger, but that's on you too. It's hard for you to be direct and clear about how hurt and angry you are. Let's hear it now."

With that, Evan started to cry. Silent tears streamed down his cheeks faster than he could wipe them away. He confided, "I just always feel like a piñata with her and her constant jabs. In high school, I felt lucky to have her – like I thought that she was better than I was too. That's not a terrible feeling in high school. It is now, though. It fucking is now. I'm not the smartest or most successful guy in the world, and now, everybody sees me as this creep, but I tried to be a good husband."

After a brief silence, I softly said, "So with each complaint, she confirmed your worst fear-that you weren't good enough for her. Seems like part of you finally said, 'Fuck it then, I'll stop trying.' Maybe the angry part of you even wanted a little payback."

Even though Evan was the one to step outside of their marriage with his sexting, it was much easier for me to feel warmly and empathic toward him. I realized how entitled, self-involved, and aggressive I found Daphne and how much difficulty I continued to have trying to like her. She reminded me of certain anxious and irritable people in my own life, and I told myself that I needed to connect more with the vulnerability underneath her abrasiveness.

To that end, the first half of my individual session with Daphne was dedicated to validating her feelings of betrayal and humiliation. She was understandably bereft and furious. Daphne had partially transferred her intense feelings of dependency from her father to Evan, and he had let her down in a traumatic way. Once she calmed down, Daphne said, "I don't see how I could ever trust him again. He broke my heart. He broke my trust. My parents are so disappointed in him too. They will never look at him the same way again. None of us will."

"It was devastating," I said, "and there is no way to sugarcoat what happened. It was a huge betrayal, but you don't have to make any decisions right now. You can give yourself time to absorb and, hopefully, understand what has happened and maybe even the reasons why."

"What is there to understand?" she challenged me. "Evan is a piece of shit, and this girl is a whore."

Though I didn't know how it would be received, I felt a need to respond and countered, "I know this is hard to hear right now, but Evan is still the same guy that you've been with since high school – the same guy that you fell in love with. He made some hurtful decisions, and I think we need to understand why before you decide what you want to do about it."

"I want to fucking kill him, that's what I want to do about it!" Daphne all but spat at me.

"I know you do," I told her. "I know you do."

During these months of estrangement from Evan, Daphne predictably leaned hard on her parents for emotional support. She worked from seven to seven, went to her parents' house for dinner, and came home in time to see Evan watching football and finishing the remnants of his fast-food dinner.

During this time, Daphne showed signs of resilience that surprised all three of us. She met with her psychiatrist, and together, they decided to increase her anti-depressant medication. She reached out to her girlfriends and made plans to go for drinks, to the movies, and even to see *Dear Evan Hanson* in the city. She began taking canasta lessons with her mother on Saturday mornings, after which the two would go to lunch at a nearby diner and talk for hours. With this new effort to take care of herself, Daphne was feeling more in control of her life, and not surprisingly, her panic attacks lessened.

In our next individual session, I talked with Daphne about how she felt growing up with her parents and her reliance on the gleam that she saw in her father's eye. She believed that her father felt she could do no wrong. Daphne lamented that she wanted her husband to feel that way about her, too, and his "going after this teenager" made her feel like she wasn't special to him at all. We explored that when Evan didn't bow to her demands, didn't follow her career advice, and didn't sacrifice himself in the wee hours of the morning to sit with her again in an emergency room, she felt like she wasn't important to him.

I also tried to help her see how she idealized her father as a strong provider and protector and often compared Evan unfavorably to him. And I encouraged her to imagine what these ongoing comparisons felt like for Evan.

This type of self-reflection didn't come easily to Daphne and was particularly difficult in the wake of Evan's betrayal. In her eyes, her demands and frequent criticism paled in comparison to his infidelity. Despite this, Daphne gradually found the courage to look at her role in the turbulence that shook her marriage.

Evan continued to sleep in the guest room for the next few months. He quickly got a job at another gym and had business cards made so he could start personal training on his own. Daphne was relieved to see him sitting in their living room when she came home at night but couldn't bear any interaction with him that smacked of normalcy. The couple spoke minimally each night, and when they did, it usually devolved into Daphne telling Evan that what he did was unforgivable and she hated him. Absent from her rantings, however, was the word "divorce," just as it was absent from our individual sessions.

When Daphne was ready, we resumed the marital sessions. I'm not sure which of the three of us was more nervous when we started again. I knew that Evan was extremely remorseful, but I also knew that if this relationship was to survive, he needed to talk about his anger and how Daphne consistently made him feel. Daphne's insecurity, her deep feelings of betrayal, and her need for more passion, intensity, and involvement from Evan also needed to be explored so that a measure of vitality could be infused into this failing relationship.

"Who would like to begin?" I asked, slightly anxious to see the direction this second first session would take.

"Let me," Evan uncharacteristically jumped in. "Daphne, you have no idea how sorry I am. I fucked up so badly. I never touched that girl – I never kissed her, I never took her out, nothing. But what I did was still awful, and I don't have any excuses."

Daphne began to cry, and through her tears, she pleaded, "But I don't understand why. I don't understand what you could have been thinking. Didn't you think about me at all?"

"I don't know what I was thinking," Evan told her. "I wasn't thinking."

"Maybe that's not the question that we need to be asking." I interjected. "Maybe the question is what have you been feeling that could have led you to do this?"

"Can I answer that, Daph? Will you listen if I answer that? Because I don't want to get you even madder at me," Evan said.

Daphne snapped back, "There's nothing you can say that will make it okay, but go ahead, what the fuck were you feeling that you had to sext with a seventeen-year-old girl?"

Evan began, "I didn't have to – I was stupid. I should have talked to you a long time ago. I should have said something in here, but part of me had already checked out. The best that I can understand is, you know how my mom constantly treats my father like he's a nothing and he can't do anything that's good enough – sometimes, that's how you make me feel. I'm not smart enough. I don't make enough money. I don't talk enough. I don't help you enough when you have your panic attacks. Your constant jabs and complaints make me feel like a loser. Then, this stupid girl made me feel like I was unbelievable – like somebody special and hot, and I won't lie – that part felt really good. I don't want to be with anyone else – ever. I just want to feel like you think I'm special and I'm good enough. I don't think I've ever felt that way with you, not since the beginning." And with that huge truth, Evan sat back in his chair and exhaled, feeling like he had just jumped off a bridge.

"Maybe I didn't think you were good enough, but I always thought that you could be good enough. I don't need you to be a doctor like my father, but I need you to be someone who goes all in to support me and take care of me and kids when we have them. You don't go all in on anything. You sit back with your video games and your quiet, and I never feel like I can really count on you. I don't know what you're thinking or feeling or planning. It just looks like you don't do anything that's hard – like you just don't want to challenge yourself. I guess you're not that guy who's all in. But I have always felt like you could be that guy if you just tried harder," Daphne told him with an energy that oozed hopefulness despite the tears in her eyes.

And there it was. With so much fear and so many swallowed emotions, I was surprised that their sex life was as good as chicken parm. Now that Evan's difficulty with anger and direct communication and his inhibited drive and ambition were out on the table, as was Daphne's underlying insecurity, her desperate need for emotional support, and her harsh defensiveness, we could begin to do the work of healing. And while we were still months away, I hoped that the healing would include each of them remembering why they loved chicken parm.

Several weeks later, I got a call from Daphne, asking for an individual session. Since our agreement was that I would meet individually with them on an as-needed basis, I cautiously agreed. In the session, Daphne told me that she had been spending a great deal of time with her mother, and the two were growing much closer. When Daphne shared with her mother that she was struggling to forgive Evan but didn't know how anyone with any self-respect could forgive such a betrayal, her mother told her that this was something she knew a little bit about. Her mother confided in her that her father had had an affair many years ago, an affair that lasted over a year and almost ended their marriage. She told her that forgiveness takes time and requires that one keep the big picture in mind. Did Daphne want to have a family and a life with Evan? Did she still love him? This news shocked Daphne but also seemed to lessen the shame that was weighing her down and holding her back.

As Daphne idealized her father less, she was able to talk about how guilty she felt that her father obviously favored her over her sister. In one session, she even wondered aloud what this was like for her older sister and guessed that it was probably very painful for her.

As she spoke, I saw the seeds of empathy begin to take root in Daphne. I watched her gradually feel remorse for chronically making Evan feel like a disappointment as a provider and as an emotional partner. She started to notice Evan's kindness and his many unique strengths. Slowly, she began to see him as a different kind of man than her father but not a lesser man.

Daphne was becoming a young woman who was able to self-reflect and tolerate uncomfortable feelings such as hurt, disappointment, and fear. She was beginning to understand her anxiety around leaving the safety and emotional protection of her parents' home and taking on the challenges of adulthood. Not surprisingly, her anxiety and panic attacks continued to lessen in both frequency and intensity.

During this time, I began to feel the warmth toward Daphne and pride in her burgeoning resilience that I had been hoping to feel.

Evan became much more communicative, letting Daphne know when she was pushing him too far and, importantly, when he was finding her particularly appealing. Their relationship seemed more playful toward the end of our work together. While Daphne was still demanding and critical, Evan handled this with humor rather than shutting down and remained engaged and available to her. I knew that they were ready to end treatment when they were each offering the other the affirming responses that they longed for. Evan said to Daphne, "You are such a tease. You were so flirting with the bartender last night."

"I wasn't really flirting with him; I was trying to make you jealous. Looks like it worked," Daphne snapped back in a feisty manner.

"Fucking right it did. I don't want anyone else near my gorgeous wife. You're mine!" Evan pronounced with all the macho assertiveness that Daphne had been craving.

Two years after we stopped working together, I got a text from Daphne. As I prepared to open the text, I worried that Evan might have acted out again or her anxiety may have gotten worse. When I clicked on the text, I was greeted with a picture of Daphne and Evan beaming, holding a beautiful little baby. Underneath the picture, she had written, "Our little cutlet."

If I Could Turn Back Time

During our work together, Daphne and Evan developed an ability to understand and empathize with each other's emotional experience and with their own age-appropriate developmental struggles around separation, individuation, and intimacy. They learned that Evan needed affirming and admiring reactions from Daphne, and they came to understand how her aggressive and demeaning comments and constant comparisons to her father made Evan feel like a failure.

Daphne began to recognize how vulnerable and furious she felt when Evan couldn't seamlessly provide the support, protection, and guidance that she had relied on her father to provide. Daphne needed Evan's calm and steady help to learn to manage her overwhelming anxiety, and she longed to feel taken care of by him as her strong and protective partner. Evan learned how his anger was manifested in his passivity and refusal to pursue goals that were in his and Daphne's best interest and, later, in his sexting with a young client. The couple eventually became able to communicate more directly about their own needs and fears, and both the emotional and sexual aspects of their relationship were reenergized.

Despite these successes, there is much I would do differently if I had the chance to do this treatment over again. I would pay more attention to my polarized experience of the couple – my feelings of dislike for Daphne and my inclination to empathize with Evan. I was aware that the intellectual, controlling, and bullying version of Daphne reminded me of several members of my own family, but I didn't fully acknowledge to myself how put off I was by the needy and anxious part of Daphne. Her utter dependence on the support and protection of others and her lack of resilience both concerned and repulsed me, as I prioritize independence and emotional fortitude in my own life.

Rather than being angered by Daphne's helplessness and externalization of responsibility for managing her anxiety, Daphne needed me to respond to her longing for a strong parental figure who could help her feel safe and understood and teach her how to manage her emotional world. If I could turn back time, I would understand these needs sooner and become the idealizable therapist that she needed me to be to a much greater extent than I did. In this way, I would have supported Daphne more as she struggled to manage disruptive feelings of anxiety and later, when she felt betrayed by Evan.

If I had it to do over again, I would look deeper into Evan's character structure and not be so quick to see him as the quiet, bullied, and beleaguered spouse. I would probe sooner for how he handled his rage as well as his identification with his father and his ambivalence around assertiveness, competition, and success.

Finally, if I could turn back time, I would follow Leone's (2021) guidance and offer Daphne more cognitive-behavioral strategies as an adjunct to our psychoanalytic couple therapy. Daphne's panic attacks were disrupting her ability to function as an adult and were destabilizing her marriage to a much greater extent than with most patients I have treated. Given the havoc her anxiety was causing in her life, I think it was a clinically indicated addition to our more analytic work. Had I incorporated teaching Daphne more cognitive-behavioral strategies to manage her anxiety, she would have been able to take greater ownership of her own mental health and would have felt a greater sense of control and personal agency in her life. Perhaps had I conceptualized teaching these strategies to Daphne as part and parcel of serving as an idealizable therapist for her, I could have done so with a fuller heart.

References

Leone, C. (2021). The application of contemporary self psychology to couple psychotherapy. *Couple and Family Psychoanalysis*, 11(2): 170–186.

5   What's That Smell?

Introduction

I tried hard not to yell as a parent. I understood firsthand how a parent's boom-ing voice, boiling with frustration and rage, could be soul crushing. When sufficiently aggravated, I would say to my kids, "I'm going to yell. Keep it up and I'm going to yell. Make sure that's what you want to happen, because if you don't start listening . . . I'm going to yell." I think they all felt, "For God's sake, just yell already!"

In the following story, you'll meet Jen, a chronically angry woman and an exceedingly difficult patient. Just keeping her engaged in treatment felt like a daunting task. My aversion to being the recipient of someone's anger and my conflict around expressing anger myself made working with her espe-cially challenging for me. Like my mother, I tended to choose brief periods of silent abandonment over outward aggression – it always felt like a "first, do no harm" tactic. Of course, neither is a good option in clinical work. My approach with Jen was to empathically consider the severe vulnerabilities underlying her rage, but this was of limited help in the face of her unrelenting hostility. Was I wrong to patiently endure her verbal assaults and prioritize creating a safe relationship in which she could bring all parts of herself and feel seen, accepted, and understood? Or should I have addressed Jen's attacks from the start, setting limits with her as we explored the triggers for her fury and the effect of her viciousness on me and others? This story considers the enactments that emerged as I navigated Jen's emotional vitriol and the devas-tating impact of my misattunement when I stopped being so careful.

What's That Smell?

"What's that smell?" Jen demanded to know as she entered my office for the first time.

"The smell?" I asked tentatively.

"The smell in your waiting room, the awful smell. You are familiar with the word, aren't you? This better not give me a migraine," she all but spat at me.

DOI: 10.4324/9781003543343-6

"Let's hope not," I said with as much sincerity as I could muster, already feeling a headache of my own coming on.

Jen was a forty-four-year-old single woman consumed with envy and rage when she began treatment with me. During much of our work together, I struggled to simply tolerate being in the room with her, and I soon realized I wasn't alone in my strong reaction. Jen and I met twice a week for seven long years. Professionally, I was focused on helping her feel understood and hoped to smooth the razor-sharp interpersonal edges with which she engaged the world. My personal focus was on staying alive and emotionally present in the face of her relentless hostility.

Jen was tall and thin, with shoulder-length light-brown hair that was often pulled back in a tight ponytail. She appeared uncomfortable in her own skin and did little to combat the plainness of her appearance. Jen came to most sessions in skinny jeans and a sweatshirt, wearing no makeup or jewelry. Her monotone, nasal voice and flat affect made it difficult to stay awake and attuned during her long obsessive monologues.

When Jen finished complaining about the smell in my office, she continued our first session, "I've had to suffer through many incompetent therapists. You came highly recommended. I hope you won't be another disappointment."

"I'll certainly do my best," I said, feeling more than a prickle of irritation almost immediately. I struggled to muster a small parcel of curiosity and asked, "Would you like to tell me about your past experiences in therapy?" I was think-ing this was what was foremost on Jen's mind and was certain that I needed to learn about my predecessors' fate and the roles I was soon to be cast in.

"Why would I want to waste my time going over other people's failures? How would that help me? Kind of a stupid question, don't you think?" Jen barked at me with a sneer.

"Fair enough," I said as I silently registered the need to ask again at the earliest opportunity. Recalibrating, I tried a different tack. "How would you like to begin?"

"I have to tell you your fucking job! Great, another winner!" she hissed.

Our treatment was five minutes old, and already, I was feeling inadequate and irritated.

I decided to see how Jen would handle humor, hoping to quell her rapidly escalating irritability. Maybe she was just anxious, I hoped, given this was our first meeting. "Wow, I've pissed you off in our first three minutes. I must be off my game today. That's a record for me," I offered.

In retrospect, I wonder if I should have taken on Jen's anger from the very beginning. While I was focused on forming a connection with her, being a container for her toxic feelings, and creating a safe space for her to express her rage, perhaps she would have benefitted from my actively engaging the angry beast in her from the start.

Jen was temporarily taken aback by my warmth and use of humor. She stopped slinging verbal arrows at me and began to talk about her childhood. Jen seemed to have a clear sense of what a good psychoanalytic patient should talk about and easily went into a practiced script about her early years. I sensed that she was emotionally stuck in these years and was eager to list her childhood grievances for a new audience.

Trading on the momentary feeling of goodwill, I tried my earlier question again. "I know I asked at the beginning of the session, but can you tell me about your past therapists – kind of a heads-up on what mistakes I should try hard not to make?"

Jen smirked and reported, "The last one was very well known. I was told he lectured all over the world. He had a very professional office – a desk and lots of books. Not like this place," she stated smugly. After glancing around my office disdainfully, Jen continued, "Really, he was a dull little man who liked to stare and wait for me to do all the work. He said next to nothing, which annoyed me, and when he did talk, he was very condescending. I wasted four years with him and finally told him to go fuck himself when he insisted that I needed to see a psychiatrist because of 'anger issues.' The therapist before him was an older woman, a complete know-it-all. She wore fancy clothes and clearly thought being a Ph.D. made her special. I think she felt threatened by my intelligence and was extremely argumentative. I saw her for two years. She was useless too. There were a few others before them. Honestly, I'm not sure why I keep trying."

I realized with this list that any attempt to challenge her defenses, understand the experiences of others, or introduce my own experience with her would need to wait until we had established a bond – if, that is, I could establish a bond with this very irritable woman.

Sensing an opportunity to end the first session on a positive note, I responded, "It's a credit to you that you keep trying. I think the understanding you are looking for in therapy is very important to you. I hope I can help you."

Over the first few months of our work together, Jen continued to tell me about her family and her struggles growing up. As the youngest of three with two older brothers, Jen was raised in a wealthy Maryland suburb just outside of D.C. Her mother was a stay-at-home mom who showed little interest in her children, especially her youngest child. Jen struggled to capture her mother's attention and never felt able to win her approval. Her mother wouldn't miss a hair appointment to pick Jen up from school when she was sick, nor would she get off a phone call to help her daughter with homework. According to Jen, her mother was vain and critical and would berate her for her lack of friends, plain appearance, and "whiny voice." Unlike Jen, her mother was very social. She prioritized her own social activities at their church, the country club, and the PTA and saved her caustic demeanor for her children. Jen was currently living with her mother, who was in her late eighties and weak from heart disease. Jen's resentment and hate were evident as she stated, "I like seeing her like this. She deserves a painful death."

I learned in our first few sessions that Jen's parents divorced when she was a junior in high school. Her father traveled often for work, and Jen believed that he cheated on his wife at every opportunity. Jen described him as a very critical man who routinely eviscerated her for her B average and lack of interest in sports, clothes, or anything else that he might have found redeeming. She reported that her father preferred her two older brothers, both of whom did well in school and were quite athletic. Her father never protected her from their teasing, and the three rarely included her in activities that they enjoyed together. Jen's father died several years after she graduated from college, leaving her feeling rejected, angry, and envious of the involved relationship he had enjoyed with her brothers.

Jen had immense difficulty sitting still and listening to authority figures throughout her childhood. Whether it was with her teacher, the bus driver, or the lunch lady, Jen was combative and noncompliant. Though teachers suggested she might be struggling with attention-deficit/hyperactivity disorder (ADHD) and would benefit from therapy and medication, Jen's parents dismissed their recommendations. "If your teacher knew how to run her classroom, we wouldn't have this problem. You just need to stop being such a brat," they admonished her.

During her high school years, Jen had only a few equally awkward friends and spent much time alone in her room. Her social isolation continued throughout her time at a small, expensive private college, where she lived in a single dorm room for all four years. Jen did not date or have any sexual experiences until the spring of her junior year of college, when she had a brief sexual encounter with a freshman boy while intoxicated. She judged football games and frat parties as "stupid wastes of time" but occasionally attended church-related events with her friend Marcy. Even there, she felt like an outsider and considered the others "losers."

Adulthood proved equally disappointing for Jen. After college, she moved in with her critical and argumentative mother and attended a local third-tier law school. Jen was still unable to form close friendships or intimate relationships, and her only consistent social contact was her older cousin Edna. The two would meet for dinner at a nearby diner every other week and lament about the multitude of injustices they each suffered growing up. When I asked more about her friendship with Edna, Jen was quick to correct me. "She's not my friend! Aren't you listening? She's my cousin. She's ugly and awkward and kind of stupid. She's not someone I would ever be friends with," Jen snapped at me.

I winced as the caustic words flowed from Jen like the rushing waters of a river. No one seemed safe from her debasement, and no one managed to touch her heart. As her bitterness washed over me, flickers of hope still sparked in my mind. *Perhaps she just needs to feel safe and understood before she can allow for any warmth or even a glimmer of trust*, I told myself.

Jen struggled through law school and required three attempts to pass the bar exam. After graduating, she spent eighteen long months searching for a job and finally secured a position at a very small firm that handled traffic ticket litigation. Jen was enraged that her new job lacked prestige and significant financial compensation. Once again, she complained that the spoils were there for others while she was unfairly shunned and denied deserved opportunities.

Despite her dissatisfaction, Jen remained at this job for more than ten years. She was finally terminated because of ongoing complaints from clients about her irritability and one very public argument she had with an older female client, around the same age as her mother. Six months after the humiliation of being fired, a depressed and extremely agitated Jen began treatment with me.

During the first few years of our work together, I felt a great deal of sadness and compassion for Jen – that is, until the moment she angrily stomped into my office every Monday and Thursday evening. I reminded myself before each session of how desperately alone she was and how demoralized she felt as she struggled to find a job in her field. Despite my emotional preparations, seeing Jen's familiar scowl at the start of each session caused my feelings of compassion to sour, and I braced myself for the onslaught of bitterness and hostility that inevitably turned up.

Jen vomited her hate and anger onto me as she spoke with disgust about her daily conflicts with her aging mother, her selfish brothers, her petty co-workers at her old job, and the "lowlifes" she encountered at her neighborhood bar. In one session a few years into our work together, Jen talked about letting a "total loser" buy her drinks on nights when they both found themselves at the bar. Jen explained, "Marv is a big fat guy. He can't get a girlfriend, so I let him buy me drinks. We watch whatever game is on and make fun of some of the assholes there. I know he wants to get with me, but that isn't happening. He's a big fat slob."

Looking to find a kernel of hope in this interaction, I asked, "Do you see him as a friend?"

Jen's nostrils flared as she angrily responded, "God no! Why would I want such a loser as a friend? He's a ticket for a few drinks. That's it!"

Jen talked about her mother's health issues, impaired mobility, and increased dependency on her that Jen wanted no part of. "She can't drive anymore and always asks me to take her here or there – a doctor's appointment, the mall, church. Fuck that! I told her she spends good money on an aide who drives, so she can use her," Jen vented.

"She wouldn't make time for you when you counted on her growing up, maybe it feels like payback," I suggested.

Feeling validated, Jen continued, "Let one of her darling sons drive her around. Just because I live in the same house with her doesn't mean I'm her chauffeur."

Jen was no more endearing with me. She often made comments such as, "Those look like very expensive shoes. I'm glad that my hard-earned money is being used for something so important" or "It's good that you don't worry about people thinking you're too old for that convertible you drive."

Her envy and resentment flowed freely in our sessions, and I often used humor to absorb the blows, manage my own anger, and hold onto my hope of reaching a less hostile side of Jen. Sometimes, when her attacks were even more direct, I held her gaze and tried to understand with her the purpose of her rage. "You get so angry with me so quickly. I wonder if you're showing me what it felt like to be you, with your mother growing up," I suggested after she criticized me for starting our session a minute and a half late. When Jen silently glared in response, I added, "And maybe you are showing yourself how powerful it can feel to be the one doing the attacking."

I considered asking Jen how she thought her comments made me feel or if she thought that I, or anyone else for that matter, had any feelings at all. Given her volatility and emotional fragility, I was concerned that Jen would either kill or crumble if she felt shamed by me. I also felt badly about how much I disliked her when she was so unrelentingly abrasive. These feelings made me feel petty and judgmental, but I was unable to shake them.

Despite my strongly mixed feelings about Jen, I very much wanted to help her feel understood and cared about in our relationship. I wanted to help her understand the very sound reasons for her rage and how she used her aggression as a protective measure to keep me and others from hurting her. I prioritized offering Jen the kind of affirming and protective emotional experiences within our relationship that she desperately needed but didn't get as a child over appealing to her intellectually with interpretations and insight. In hindsight, I wonder whether addressing her rage and envy more directly might have been more effective in helping her feel seen, understood, and impactful.

While Jen was very unlike the people in my world, the frequent bursts of anger and criticism that she directed at me were all too familiar. My mind drifted in one session to when I was ten, stuck in holiday traffic and sandwiched between my older brother and sister in the back seat of our old brown Oldsmobile Cutlass. Though I knew it was a bad idea, I couldn't stop myself from asking my father why he had chosen that route home. The car suddenly erupted with his anger, as if my question broke the concentration that he needed to simply keep the car on the road. Another time, my thoughts drifted back to my brother's mocking taunts at the dinner table, delivered in hushed whispers and aimed with laser-like precision at my most acute insecurity of the moment. As these memories skated across my consciousness in sessions, I realized how bullied I felt by Jen, just as I had at times in my family growing up.

Despite her haughty and hostile demeanor, I continued to search for the strength and kernels of good in Jen. I reminded myself that she never experienced feelings of admiration or encouragement from her parents and that their constant criticism taught her only how to condemn. I hoped that by magnifying the tendrils of humor and kindness she sparingly showed, I could help her feel seen and appreciated for her warmer, more engaging side. I believed this would help build her self-esteem, expand her view of herself in a more positive way, and help her experience less exclusively toxic interactions with the others. Selfishly, I longed for even a brief reprieve from her disdain and the frequent criticism that was consistently directed my way.

During one session, several years into our work together, Jen was being uncharacteristically funny while discussing politics. Wanting to share my delight in her knowledge and how amusing she could be, I said, "You are quite well informed about politics. Talking about it seems to bring out your amusing, dry sense of humor."

"I am not paying you so I can entertain you,'" she seethed in response.

Taken aback, I countered, "You are so used to being at odds with people – it feels safer than having them or me actually enjoy parts of your personality."

"Why would I care if you enjoyed my personality? I pay you to listen to me. I couldn't care less what you find funny. That is one of the stupidest things you have said to me," she blasted me.

I let her hostile words fill the room while I met her challenging glare.

After a long silence, I said, "You're pretty hard on me. I think you use your anger to push me away and to protect yourself. Feeling alone, you can handle. Feeling hurt by someone you let close to you, not so much."

"Is that the best you've got?" Jen countered defensively.

"Might just be," I said, feeling the sense of worthlessness and futility that was all too familiar to both of us.

Despite the difficulty that Jen's case presented, I steadfastly avoided talking about her in my peer-supervision group. I eventually realized that I was working tirelessly to avoid feeling the anger and hate that she provoked in me. I dissociated my own rageful feelings to maintain my image of myself as a benevolent and competent therapist. By shutting down my anger, I quieted this conflict and addressed my fear that I would hurt Jen should I allow myself to fully experience my rage. While this dissociation helped me manage our relationship over the long haul, I was less emotionally honest and authentically present with Jen as a result. It also denied her the experience of our addressing the ruptures that her relentless attacks provoked and the *in vivo* repair of our relationship.

There were occasional moments when Jen experienced me as the warm and caring mother she longed for as a child. She proudly showcased her organizational talent and slowly developing interpersonal skills as she spoke in detail about the freelance work she was doing for a small eldercare law firm. In doing so, Jen looked to me as an encouraging, approving parent who could help her enjoy feelings of pride and personal success.

Similarly, she shared her attempts at exercise and healthy eating as she knew, through tidbits I had shared, that these were interests of mine. Jen basked in my eagerness to hear about her experiences at the gym, including her preference for spin class over yoga and her occasional sessions with a young, handsome personal trainer. I also asked questions about the new recipes she occasionally mentioned trying and nodded with understanding when she lamented that these dishes were prepared for an audience of one.

More often, I was experienced as the critical, rejecting mother of her childhood, and I was emotionally eviscerated by Jen. I was told I was of "mediocre intelligence" and called money hungry and self-indulgent. She insisted that

I charged an exorbitant fee because I was greedy and ended sessions early because I was lazy. I was a privileged, entitled, self-involved woman – just like her mother. During these times, Jen would experience almost any question, comment, or attempt to help her focus on a particular issue as criticism. She would stare at the clock when I spoke as if each syllable was torturous and responded to my few words with accusations and insults.

During one session three years into our work together, I commented, "I noticed that you tend to stare at the clock when I talk."

"I'm just seeing how much of my time you are going to waste. You like to hear yourself talk," Jen said, looking me straight in the eyes and sneering.

I was experiencing that familiar sense of being bullied by her and felt that several years into the treatment, this bitter, emotionally terrified woman could tolerate a little more pushback.

We had talked often about how similar she felt I was to her mother and her expectation that like her mother's, my words would burn with criticism and contempt. With this in mind, I asked, "It's so much safer for you to assume that I'm just like your mother, that I don't care about you. Is it possible that occasionally, I might say something helpful, something that might make you feel understood, even important to me?"

Jen swallowed hard and looked up at me. I saw an eight-year-old girl desperate for recognition and affection and felt an uncomfortable urge to give her a hug. I understood both of our reactions as a sign that this need/fear dilemma around emotional closeness was at the heart of Jen's struggle.

I also realized that the rage she directed at me was not simply rooted in her expecting/re-experiencing her mother's utter lack of attunement, criticism, and callous dismissal. When I sat silently, listening and absorbing her fury, I was a safe harbor where she could seek respite and protection from a world of hostile others. Perhaps she even imagined my solidarity with her in her battles. But when I spoke, the magical spell was broken. I became a separate person, another tormenter, destined to misunderstand and despise her.

There were many days when I questioned whether I was the best analyst for Jen. Some days, when her verbal attacks were particularly vicious, I felt too sensitive and too vulnerable to effectively stave off her onslaughts. I imagined the clock moving backward as she would drone on about my or someone else's many shortcomings, and occasionally, my mind silently screamed, "SHUT THE FUCK UP!"

At these times, I told myself that my work with Jen was my penance for having a large caseload of warm, grateful patients who fed my need to feel helpful and appreciated. This explanation, however, was incomplete. Despite her near-constant aggressiveness, I felt a sense of caring and warmth for her. There was a certain sassiness in her combativeness that sometimes made me smile. I very much wanted to push through her barbed-wire defenses and help her find some relief from her emotional suffering. Jen had lived the bulk of her life with a self-absorbed, inattentive mother who was irritated by her normal developmental needs. She deserved an analytic mother who would be there for her, putting her own needs for emotional respite on the back burner. And so the dance between my heartfelt wish to heal and my human wish for self-protection went on.

During the final months of our work together, Jen's mother became increasingly ill, and Jen faced an aloneness that chilled me to the bone. Her alcohol and pill use increased dramatically, as did the intensity of her conflicts with her brothers and friends of the family around their mother's care and finances. When I shared my deep concern about her increased use of alcohol and prescription medication, Jen was furious. She couldn't feel the concern in my voice and heard only criticism and condemnation in my words.

As the prospect of her mother's death loomed, Jen became increasingly volatile and experienced me almost exclusively as the self-serving, critical mother of her childhood. During one session, she recounted spending a long evening eating and drinking at the bar she frequented. Jen described taking a Valium hours earlier, after her oldest brother infuriated her by criticizing how she spent money. Even more enraging, he doubted her ability to handle the sizable amount of money that she would soon inherit. Once at the bar, Jen began drinking vodka and club sodas while watching the football game with Marv and a few of the other regulars. A disgusted Jen explained that five hours and six or seven drinks later, Marv tried to kiss her. She screamed at him and threw a drink in his face. At this point, the "asshole" bartender took her car keys and insisted that she needed to leave and should take an Uber home.

Jen was in a rage as she recounted her predicament; she could either create a scene in the only place that offered her respite from her isolation, or she could "demean" herself and agree to call an Uber. Jen chose the latter, but not without whispering to the bartender, "I won't forget this you faggot! You and this fat fuck will be sorry you turned on me."

Feeling like I was navigating in a minefield but wanting to highlight how things seemed to be spinning out of control, I responded, "Wow, sounds like that got awful fast. How do you understand how that all unfolded?"

Jen snapped, "Marv is a pig, and James is an asshole bartender who hates women – that's it."

As I tried to explore the role of her increased drinking and the trouble that she was narrowly escaping because of it, Jen built a case in her own mind that I was attacking her, just like her mother. Jen raged at me, "You think you're so high and mighty and I'm a nothing. You want to make it like it's my fault so you can tell me what I did wrong. Sorry to tell you, but I think you're pathetic. You don't know the first thing about me or what I'm dealing with."

The following week, Jen was unusually late for our session. I found myself walking into the waiting room feeling a medley of annoyance and concern. While Jen's lateness was a recent development, missing almost half the session was unprecedented in our work together. As I walked back into my office, Jen stormed in. Finding me standing, she blurted out in an accusatory manner, "Where are you going?"

"I was just walking around. I was concerned about you. You are unusually late," I responded.

Jen snapped in an irritated tone, "I highly doubt that! You were probably looking to leave early and get out of doing any work. Not that what you do should count as work anyway."

Though irritated, I calmly said, "Would it be crazy to think that I'm concerned about you?"

Jen responded, "I am not here to talk about you. You have wasted enough of my time," and then launched a typical rant vilifying her brother and sister-in-law.

Jen's lateness reflected her overwhelming anxiety around her mother's impending death and her desperate need for a modicum of control as she felt her small world unraveling. In the final weeks of our work together, Jen was arriving twenty to thirty minutes late to sessions. These sessions became increasingly difficult to end on time because she would remain seated and ignore my prompts to wind down. During one of our last sessions, I had to repeat several times that we needed to stop, eventually standing and walking toward the door. "Jen, we really have to stop for today. We can take our time talking about this next week," I assured her in my third attempt to get her to leave my office.

"All you care about is yourself. You like having all the power. I can't always operate on other people's time schedules. You really are incredibly selfish!" she defiantly scolded me. Jen kept talking as she reluctantly walked out of my office. She was detailing how useless our sessions were and questioning whether she should just stop coming while walking through the waiting room. She became even more enraged when I told her we couldn't continue to talk in this very public area and I would see her in a few days.

In the next session, I discussed with Jen that while she had recently been very late to sessions, she was also having tremendous difficulty leaving when our time was up. Perhaps, I suggested, at such a difficult time in her life, she felt that she needed me and our time together but found this need more uncomfortable than either of us had anticipated. It wasn't until a few days later, when I received her barrage of vicious messages ending the treatment, that I realized my misattuned exposure of her dependency on me had unintentionally delivered a humiliating blow.

It was an unremarkable Monday morning when I checked my work phone to gear up for the week ahead. I lost my breath as I listened to an avalanche of threatening voicemails from Jen that had been sent steadily since the night before. "I am done with you! You have been a huge disappointment to me. You don't listen. You don't pay attention. You are the worst fucking therapist in the world. You have taken advantage of me for the last time. Never contact me again, or you will regret it." The disdain and viciousness in her voice left me feeling frightened and sick.

By the sixth or seventh voicemail, Jen reiterated that she would not be returning to treatment and that I was not to call or text her again. In the last message, she told me that I should be afraid and that she was not a person to be trifled with. A stream of similarly hateful and threatening voicemails was sent over the next several days.

The Monday-morning onslaught caught me by surprise. I knew Jen was reeling from the impending loss of her mother and had been drinking more and taking prescription pills. She was enraged by the increased contact with her older brothers around their mother's imminent death and what she saw as their critical and controlling attitude toward her. I knew that I would be the target of much of Jen's anger, but I didn't anticipate the violent mauling of the therapeutic bond. I was left replaying our last few sessions, wondering how I tripped through her looking glass and wound up in the graveyard of hated former therapists. I was left examining my role in the rupture that incited this brutal ending to our work together.

At first, it seemed that this long and painful treatment died a rather sudden death amid a flurry of threats and accusations. In retrospect, I don't believe it was sudden at all. With her mother's death looming, Jen felt even more dependent on me, and these feelings of dependency felt deadly to her. While she was always guarded against any experience of emotional need or longing, she was now unable to tolerate anything or anyone that threatened further loss. It was kill or be killed in Jen's roguish internal world. As she battered me and our relationship with her lateness and her heightened combativeness, I believe that I finally succumbed and delivered the humiliation that she had both invited and feared since our first moments together.

Several weeks after Jen left treatment, I sent her the following note detailing the progress I felt she had made in our work together that I hoped would be healing. "I so appreciate that you let me into your life. You very bravely shared with me the tremendous pain and difficult struggles that you have been through. You have come a long way in being able to understand and talk about your feelings, even in realizing the ways in which you sometimes push away relationships you might benefit from. I know that my ability to help you has reached its limit, but I do hope you continue in treatment. To that end, I have included the names of two very experienced therapists who I think would be a good fit. I wish you the best."

I got a text from Jen several months later telling me that her mother had died. "I certainly don't want to talk to you again," she wrote. "I just thought that you would want to know."

I was heartened to learn that I was no longer living in Jen's mind as purely selfish and hurtful and that she was able to think of me as caring about her as well. I texted back, "I am so sorry to hear that. I can only imagine how difficult this time must be for you. Thank you for letting me know about your mom. Please take care of yourself."

Three months later, I received a voicemail from Jen stating that she was beginning treatment with a male therapist she had found, as she had little faith in my judgment about who she would do well with. She demanded that I contact this person and fill him in on our work together. Her last words were,

"By the way, I'm doing much better without all of your overpriced help, but you weren't the worst therapist I've ever had."

I beamed at Jen's parting gift: news that she was well, delivered with her version of human kindness.

If I Could Turn Back Time

When I think about my work with Jen, I realize that simply keeping her engaged in treatment for seven long years was a therapeutic feat. While it is easy, even cathartic for me to help the highly anxious or severely depressed patient, the acting-out adolescent, or even the feuding couple, this chronically rageful woman challenged my view of myself as a caring and skilled professional. I continue to question why I fought so hard to keep Jen in treatment given how toxic and painful I found our sessions to be. I know I felt a responsibility to provide some of the protective functions and emotional supplies that Jen needed but didn't receive as a child. And I know that I wanted to ease her near-constant emotional suffering. But I realize that I also needed to protect my view of myself as a clinician who can reach the exceedingly difficult patient and survive in the stormiest therapeutic waters.

First, if I could turn back time, here's what I would not change. While many would suggest that Jen needed firm limits set regarding her frequent personal insults and attacks, I felt that invoking the power of my position by doing so would have been a mistake. I believed that Jen needed me to experience over and over what she endured as a child. How else could I truly know the feelings of powerlessness that she experienced and the rage that was her response to this chronic and destabilizing feeling? Jen was a fighter, and while her aggression was often extreme and misdirected, this fire was also key to her emotional survival.

If I could turn back time, I would highlight the adaptive purpose or the forward edge (Tolpin, 2002) of her relentless aggression more often and more clearly than I did. I wish I would have said something like, "Jen, becoming a fighter was one way to make sure you never felt as powerless as you felt growing up. Your anger helps you feel stronger and tells the world that you won't be treated poorly." This could have helped her feel understood and might have mitigated the deep shame that festered within her.

Given Jen's anticipation of crushing criticism and her deep fear of connection, I took great care to protect her fragile self-esteem and highly reactive defenses – that is, until I didn't. I wondered about my role in the fatal rupture, when I highlighted Jen's dependency on me at such a painful time in her life. I wondered why I chose then to be so direct.

If I could turn back time, I would be more in touch with the enactment that Jen and I were engaged in when her mother's death became imminent. While I was aware that Jen was pushing me away as her fear of loss and feelings of need intensified, I was not aware of how I dissociated my own emotional response to her mother's impending death. Months after our treatment ended,

I realized how this triggered my anxiety about my mother's advanced age and health concerns. Perhaps a part of me needed to push Jen away before her mother passed – before confronting the reality of maternal loss became inescapable.

Jen's treatment highlights the importance of choosing, in select moments, between responding from within the patient's experience or from the relational "other-centered" perspective (Fosshage, 2003a; Steiner (1994). Jen presented an ongoing dilemma in this regard given her long history of emotional neglect and misattunement. My empathic, patient-centered responses often triggered both her longing for and her dread of closeness, and she would react with rage and distrust. On the other hand, reminders of my separateness and anything that smacked of prioritizing the needs or feelings of others also triggered her distrust and anger.

If I could turn back time, I would take more of a relational approach with Jen and risk being experienced as the narcissistic mother of her childhood. I would spend more time judiciously sharing my own emotional experience in the room with her and discussing the impact that she had on me and important others in her life. For example, when she told me that my red pants looked tacky and cheap, I could have responded, "Ouch! How do you imagine that makes me feel?" I might have even added, "That hurt. And it kind of felt like something your mother might have said to you."

In hindsight, my equanimity in the face of her relentless viciousness may have felt anything but empathic. My calm may have made Jen feel that her rage was ineffectual and unimportant to me. And my lack of genuine, affect-laden responses may have made me seem, like her parents, emotionally unavailable to her. By letting her see that her words could hurt or anger me and that together, we could repair each conflict, I would have been offering Jen a new kind of interpersonal experience. In this new relational dynamic, her power would be acknowledged, interpersonal consequences would be explored, and communication and forgiveness could become possible.

References

Fosshage, J.L. (2003a). Contextualizing self psychology and relational psychoanalysis: Bi-directional influence and proposed synthesis. *Contemporary Psychoanalysis*, 39: 411–448.

Steiner, J. (1994). Patient-centered and analyst-centered interpretations: Some implications of containment and countertransference. *Psychoanalytic Inquiry*, 14: 406–422.

Tolpin, M. (2002). Doing psychoanalysis of normal development: Forward edge transferences. *Progress in Self Psychology*, 18: 167–190.

6   An Unspoken Promise

Introduction

When I was a child, my mother was my favorite person. She was extremely loving and patient with me, but when she did get angry, she would give me "the silent treatment." Though it didn't happen often and rarely lasted long, I found it far more upsetting than my father's yelling. Years later, as a clinician, I have a much easier time with a patient's rage or ceaseless anxiety than with their silence.

I felt lost when I tried, session after session, to reach fourteen-year-old Mandy, and she refused to offer more than an occasional reply to my questions and quizzical looks. My inability to deeply understand what was troubling her or ease her suffering left me feeling incompetent. "An Unspoken Promise" is the story of my challenging and, at times painful work with Mandy. During our three years of work together, Mandy's longing for understanding battled her fear of closeness with me. As an unconscious compromise, we met weekly, but our time together was mostly without words.

An Unspoken Promise

"Mandy's not a troublemaker, she's a good girl," Rita insisted as she described her youngest of three children. "She's smart and has a heart of gold. She's just always so unhappy. She never wants to leave her room, and lately, she refuses to go to school. Mandy doesn't have many friends, and she won't talk to me or her sisters. She chats a little with her father but not about anything important. The more I try to find out what's going on, the more she pulls away. I don't know what to do. I leave early because I work in the city, and her father can't get her to go to school. I'm worried she's going to get left back."

Hoping to calm her mother's palpable concern and feelings of futility, I took a deep breath and responded, "I can see how hard this is for you. It's quite possible that Mandy is giving as much as she can right now. We may need to be exceptionally patient with her." We were ten minutes into the consultation, and I was already trying to lower both her mother's expectations and my own.

DOI: 10.4324/9781003543343-7

Her parents explained that Mandy had been "unhappy" as far back as either parent could remember. Rita was a high-powered Manhattan attorney who worked fourteen-hour days and hobbled home to her sleeping children each night. I would learn that Mandy found her mother demanding and irritable, and she almost automatically spurned her mother's attempts at closeness or conversation. Rita was worried, hurt, and often angry, as she found her daughter completely unreachable.

Ron, Mandy's dad, was a shy, quiet man. He had a small graphic design business and worked from home. Ron described a loving relationship with Mandy but felt unable to pry her from her room or tunnel through the walls of her depression. Despite his emotional reserve, he, Mandy, and her middle sister, Madeline, had dinner in front of the TV together every night. Seventeen-year-old Madeline would chat frenetically as Mandy and their dad sat quietly, longing for silence.

Madeline tried to navigate Mandy's withdrawal and compensate for her long silences. She was the artistic one in the family who I sensed was fighting her own very different battle with depression. Mandy's oldest sister Dalia was seven years her senior and left for college in LA when Mandy was eleven. Much like her mother, Dalia was ambitious and had little patience for Mandy's difficulty expressing herself or her chronic withdrawal.

Ron informed me that this would be Mandy's fourth stint in therapy and warned that she barely spoke to the first three therapists. The first therapist played Candyland and Scrabble with her and rarely pressed Mandy to speak. More recently, the two other therapists gave up after several sessions filled with protracted silences and unanswered questions. Like his wife, Ron was very worried by Mandy's unremitting depression and social isolation. They feared that this treatment, like those before it, would end in resounding defeat. Although withdrawn teenagers have never been my strong suit, I liked these parents very much and had the strong sense that I would like Mandy as well. *Challenge accepted*, I thought to myself.

Mandy walked into my office for our first session and stood in the middle of the room, examining her choice of seats. After careful consideration, she sat in the middle seat of the couch and rather formally said, "Hello."

"Hello," I responded. Encouraged by what seemed to be her very intense and direct manner, I continued, "So, what brings you here?"

Mandy paused for a full minute, which felt like an hour, and then said, "My parents. I have no interest in this – nothing personal, of course."

"Got it. I appreciate your honesty," I responded. "Any idea why they want you to come to therapy?" I asked.

After another very long pause, Mandy offered, "My depression," and then sat back silently.

The session was about five minutes old, and already I was getting that restless feeling, like I was trying too hard, talking too much, even breathing too loudly.

Careful not to rush her or push too hard, I sat with Mandy in silence, taking in her downward glance and the childlike way she kicked her sneakers together as she sat. After a few minutes, I nonchalantly asked, "Can you tell me about your depression?"

Mandy paused and then responded, "Nope."

"That's okay," I said. "We can take our time getting to know each other." While my brain was compiling a list of questions that couldn't easily be batted away with one-word answers, my gut told me to stop thinking and talking and simply sit with Mandy – a concept that was well outside of my very verbal comfort zone.

I noted that Mandy appeared younger than her fourteen years of age. Just over five feet tall with an athletic build, she had pale-blond hair and deep blue eyes. Mandy had huge dimples which, on the rare occasion that she smiled, made her look far happier than she felt. She also had an unusually small pinky finger on her left hand that she often covered with her other hand, a barely noticeable birth defect that she felt a need to hide. Whether it was her relentless study of the floor or the narrowing of her eyes when she dared to glance up, the message was clear: contact, never mind closeness, might be longed for but was far too terrifying to entertain.

Over the next few sessions, I asked well-paced questions about school, friends, and social activities, none of which got a response beyond "no" or "I'm not interested." When I tripped over the topic of animals, however, Mandy spoke with a surprising richness about her interest in birds. She enjoyed researching birds – where different species could be found, their unique characteristics, and what they required to flourish.

I smiled, as I was happy to hear her speak and considered that a bird seemed a perfect metaphor for Mandy's fragile and frightened self.

Suddenly, whether she saw the delight in my eyes as she spoke or noticed the enthusiasm infusing her words, Mandy pulled back and abruptly stopped talking. Her withdrawal felt like the cold slap of an icy wind and left me wondering why my visible appreciation of her felt so utterly terrifying.

Several months into our work together, Mandy was also willing to speak complete sentences about her depression. "I've always wanted to die, ever since I was little," she stated as a matter of fact. She quickly added, "That doesn't mean I'm going to kill myself. I'm not. It just means that I wish I was dead. Those other stupid therapists couldn't understand the difference."

I responded, "I want you to be able to talk with me about those feelings as often as you can. I will ask a few dumb questions, but I'll try not to jump to any conclusions, and I'll always check out what I'm thinking with you." I tried to give Mandy the feeling of control I sensed she needed. Then, I sat quietly, hoping for a response, and slowly realized that Mandy had given me her quota of words for the day.

I considered asking Mandy why she stopped talking. I thought about asking what it was like when I and everyone else in her world always wanted more from her. I even had fleeting thoughts of sharing with Mandy that she intimidated me and I was afraid that if I pushed too hard, she would abandon me. I settled for saying, "I can feel how tough it is for you to talk with me. We can just spend some time together."

Mandy's closed lips twitched, and she met my gaze for just a second.

In another session, I asked, "You mentioned that you have always wished you were dead. Can you tell me why?"

"There's a lot that I hate about myself," Mandy answered. "I'm fat. I don't have friends. I'm not like other kids. I know that I'm not normal."

"Wow, that's quite a list," I said, certain that any attempts to talk her out of this harsh assessment would be rebuffed. "How would you like to be different?" I asked.

The long silence that followed told me that once again, Mandy was done answering my questions.

Uncomfortable with leaving so much of her self-hate on the table, I asked, "Can I tell you what I think?"

"If you have to," Mandy responded, her way of granting me permission.

"You're right, you are not at all like other kids. From what I can tell so far, some of the difference is because of your depression – how little energy you have for things and how it affects the way you see yourself. Part of it, though, is who you are. You have a depth and a sensitivity and, yes, a sadness that most kids your age don't have, and you feel uncomfortable with typical kid stuff. It's like you're on a different wavelength. But that doesn't make you less wonderful." I knew that Mandy was uncomfortable with admiration, but I was determined to slowly challenge that, one carefully placed comment at a time.

Mandy looked down while I spoke, and I could feel the battle between her bittersweet longing to be seen and understood and her terror of taking in my words. Why any closeness was so terrifying to her was still unclear to me.

Eventually, Mandy began to offer me snippets about her relationship with her mother. She felt that her mother always wanted something from her that she couldn't understand, never mind provide. She described her mother's relentless questioning, which left her feeling inadequate and exhausted. Mandy found some comfort in the presence of her quiet father, who rarely pressed her to talk and didn't seem to care how she was performing, either at school or with other kids.

After a phone call from Rita in which she described Mandy as particularly "reclusive," I asked, "Can you tell me about what it's like with your mom these days?"

After several minutes of silence, Mandy replied quietly and somewhat predictably, "It's fine."

"Humor me," I said trying to sound playful. "Paint a picture for me of a typical weekend with her, maybe even last weekend," I asked, feeling that she could handle my gentle prodding.

After her trademark long silence, Mandy began to speak. "It's kind of like we are from different planets, and I can't breathe on her planet."

After a moment, I said "Wow. That's a great picture. Can you tell me about your planet?"

"No," Mandy responded unusually quickly, and I could feel the invisible but by now familiar wall go up between us.

Finally, with just a few moments left in the session, I said, "I wonder if you feel that way with me too – that you may have trouble breathing on my planet and are more than a little afraid to have me on your planet."

Mandy looked up and held my gaze. The longing for understanding that I saw in her eyes made words unnecessary, and I could feel our connection begin to deepen.

These moments of felt connection, however, were few and far between. While I tried to appear patient and self-assured, I often felt incompetent and frustrated when Mandy sat silently for most of many sessions or gave mono-syllabic responses for forty-five minutes at a time. I wanted to offer her a rela-tionship in which she could reveal the hidden sides of herself: the terrified, lonely little girl, the needy child, and the angry teenager. And I desperately wanted to be the one therapist who could find a way through her defenses and meaningfully connect with her. I didn't want to fail, for Mandy or for myself.

Despite my determination, I found myself getting frustrated, even angry at the glacially slow pace of our sessions. Suddenly, in one long and silent session, I remembered an incident when I was nine years old. I was alone at a local schoolyard, hitting a tennis ball against the building's wide wall and pretending to be in the third set of a match at Wimbledon, when a man in a white van called me over. The dark-haired, bearded driver playfully shouted, "Hey, come here. Come in the van. I have something I want to show you."

I remember standing, frozen in place, my curiosity battling my apprehension.

"Come in," he prodded with a smile. "I won't hurt you."

I slowly approached the passenger-side door, peered in the open window, and noticed an odd smell – like my father's cigars but different. Then I saw that his pants were open, and one of his hands had disappeared inside them.

"No" I said, "I can't. I'm not allowed." Suddenly, very frightened, I started backing up.

And then he was screaming, "Get the fuck out of here, then! If you come back, I'll kill you. Do you hear me? I'll kill you!"

Clutching my racquet, I ran and ran. I didn't stop until I reached my house, out of breath and out of tears. I didn't speak of this terrifying morning for over fifteen years. With this recovered memory, I felt a fresh wave of empathy for Mandy and her need to hold and protect her pain.

A year into the treatment, Mandy was experiencing a strong negative maternal transference with me. She seemed to be experiencing me as like her mother, demanding that she produce for my own satisfaction and invari-ably finding her inadequate. I believe Mandy felt I didn't appreciate the effort required for her to put her feelings into words and that she simply lacked the energy to do so. She seemed to find my constant requests to be exhausting and utterly depleting. As with her mother, she anticipated that frustration, anger, and ultimately rejection would be my certain response to her. While I hoped to make her feel valued for her simple willingness to be with me, I realized that my frequent questions suggested otherwise.

During one long and quiet session, Mandy seemed to sense that we both needed the teaspoon of hope that her audible words would offer, and she shared a dream with me. "I had a dream last night," she remarked and then leaned back in her chair.

I waited for her to continue and, when no further words were offered, I took my cue. "Can you tell me about it?" I asked.

"I'm not going to say that and then not tell you about it," she chirped, exuding a feistiness that she correctly sensed I very much enjoyed.

I, too, sat back with a slight smile and waited for the small treasure that she promised.

"I was with my friend Raina, and she was drawing with colored chalk on my driveway. I wanted to draw with her, but I didn't. I was worried that my mother was going to come home, even though I knew she wasn't coming home till much later. I wanted to tell her to stop drawing, that I was going to get in trouble, but I just stood there."

Again, I waited, taking care not to impose my pace on Mandy. When it was clear that no further details were forthcoming, I selected my questions carefully. "How do you understand the dream?"

Mandy looked like she was about to speak and then paused. After about sixty long seconds, which felt more like sixty minutes, Mandy offered, "My mom is always gonna be mad at me. I always disappoint her." As if she had been speaking for an hour, Mandy stopped talking with a sigh and studied the floor in her usual manner.

"Go on," I said, pretending that she would continue simply because I had asked her to.

"We were just going to draw. It was no big deal. I wanted to draw, but I felt like I shouldn't, and I couldn't tell Raina not to draw. I just stood there like an idiot," she added, much to my surprise.

"How do you understand the chalk?" I asked.

"I used to like to do that, I guess. It's just a stupid dream," Mandy almost whispered.

As I thought about the dream, I understood how stuck Mandy was feeling. I let this experience wash over me and finally offered, "You are in quite a bind. I think you feel like you are betraying your mother – like she will be angry with you if you 'play' with me – if you talk with me about how things are for you. But part of you wants to."

And with that interpretation, Mandy closed the portal of communication, returning to her solitary perch.

I wondered if her retreat was her idiosyncratic response to feeling understood, like one of the birds she studied, taking this morsel of understanding somewhere safe to examine it more closely. Or was it her response to the feeling of dread that understanding and closeness triggered in her? Either way, I believed that the dream was Mandy's offering to me – her quiet plea that I not give up on her. At least that was how I chose to understand it.

Rita emailed every few weeks to keep me informed about Mandy's progress in school and functioning at home, both of which were showing gradual improvement. It was in one of these emails that she told me about Ron's health problems and that tests, scans, and doctor visits were filling their days. Within weeks, Rita informed me that Ron had been diagnosed with lung cancer, and surgery and aggressive chemotherapy were scheduled. The modifier "stage 4" had been used, and a bottomless terror gripped this family. Mandy had been told of her father's illness but not its severity or the depth of their concern.

Following the surgery, her sisters came home to see their dad, and a nurse moved in to help with his care. Amid the heartbreak and commotion, and with her father's death looming, Mandy had a birthday. Ron's tender celebration of past birthdays was a painful memory. Now, he was heavily sedated and unable to leave his bed. Her mother, sisters, and visiting relatives were all preoccupied, laboring tirelessly to soften this brutal goodbye. They had little energy left to challenge Mandy's quiet withdrawal. They had little energy left to notice Mandy at all.

It was during this time that I felt my heart break. It broke for Ron, who lay dying in a hospital bed, perched where a coffee table should have been, in the middle of their living room. Through his pain and narcotic haze, I imagined him riddled with every parent's greatest terror: being unable to protect one's child, already fragile and feeling alone in the world. My heart broke for Rita, losing her partner, a man whose quiet strength she had relied on for over two decades. I felt terribly sad for Mandy's sisters and elderly grandparents, who felt shattered by the impending loss of this gentle, loving man. Most of all, my heart fell to pieces for Mandy, who tried to skirt the edges of the deep abyss that depression and loss relentlessly pulled her toward.

I wanted to take Mandy home, fix up a room for her, and chase the ghost of loss from her eyes. I wanted to at least see her more frequently, help her survive this trauma, and reassure her that she didn't have to soldier through this hell alone. Mandy refused more sessions and dismissed my offer to be available via email, phone, or text between sessions. While she would answer factual questions about her dad's condition or what was going on at home, there was no sharing of pain and no allowance for tears or laying bare her worries about the future.

The mother in me felt a desperate need to "do something." While Mandy may have grown accustomed to the depth of her pain and isolation, I had not. I wanted her to feel seen, even celebrated, despite the despair that filled her home. Given Mandy's withdrawal in and out of sessions and my vague recollection that adoption was out of the question, I settled for the only thing I felt I could do: I bought Mandy a birthday present.

My birthday gift to Mandy was a small birdhouse, notable more for its charm than its utility. When I offered the wrapped gift, announcing that I had a birthday present for her, Mandy's manner became crisp. "A birthday present," she repeated with eyes wide and a voice louder than I had heard before.

"Yes," I said. "I saw it, and I thought of you," I added, failing to mention the hours I spent online looking for a gift that she might embrace.

She carefully unwrapped the package and, acting more like a young child than a withdrawn teenager, she seemed to relish getting the gift as much as the gift itself.

The remainder of the session almost floated on her momentary emotional availability. A naive part of me hoped that we had found our way to new shores, where I could offer and Mandy could receive. A second voice warned that there would be a price to pay for these moments of unabashed warmth and closeness. I silently prayed that it wouldn't be too costly.

In hindsight, I think that this gift was my way of "doing something," of smuggling a part of myself across the barrier that Mandy always kept between us. As a transitional object, I hoped the gift would allow Mandy to feel my presence in the darkness of her day-to-day life. I imagined that when she felt especially sad and alone, she could look at the birdhouse and feel the love and concern that was an unspoken part of our relationship. I also hoped that the birdhouse would be a symbol for Mandy of being known by me and appreciated for who she uniquely was.

The next few sessions were marked by Mandy's typical lack of eye contact and terse responses. The wall was back, and I felt the wonder of connection that we so briefly shared slipping from my grasp. I learned during this time that Ron was failing rapidly. An ugly and harsh death was steaming over this man who, not so long ago, had been full of life. Mandy did not miss a session, though her words became fewer, and her subtle glances were fewer still. I will never know if my gift would have created a passable gap in the wall between us had Mandy not lost the centerpiece of her emotional world. But life's cruel turn prompted Mandy to retreat even further, and I could feel the dull ache of her loneliness become the sharpest of pain.

The months following her father's death were filled with her consistent refusal to respond to my gentle probes. For me, it was months of feeling invisible and interchangeable with the other faceless adults who were trying to comfort Mandy. Where there used to be brief responses and occasional intellectual banter, there was now only polite refusal to consider questions. "I'm not interested in talking about it," she would say.

Sometimes, I would discuss my concerns or share flashes of my experience in the room with her. These offerings were not responded to, and I was left feeling useless and exposed.

At the start of our third year together, Mandy asked, as if she needed my permission, if she could stop coming to therapy. She was unwilling to explore why now or what she imagined our stopping would mean to either of us.

I ended the session by grasping for the sliver of power that she offered me. "This is too important to decide quickly," I said. "Let's both think about it during the week and talk about it in our next session."

During the next week, I struggled mightily with my ambivalence about my work with Mandy. While my feelings of love and compassion ran deep for this sixteen-year-old girl, so too did the feelings of rejection and uselessness that I felt in the dark shade of her wall. I kept summoning myself back to what I felt she needed most from me at this crossroads. Was it recognition of her ability to walk through the treacherous sands of her depression while meeting the minimal demands of each day? Was it support for the teenager that she was becoming and for the voice she raised in asking for this separation? Or did she need me to hold on tight as her single point of connection while she struggled to metabolize her father's death and find the will to inch forward?

The following week's session opened with a long stretch of silence as the threat of mutual loss hung heavy in the air between us. Finally, I asked Mandy if she had thought more about what she brought up the week before.

"I don't think I need to come here," she said firmly. "I am going to school. I am doing what I have to do. Nothing personal," she added with a quick glance, and I saw the slightest crack in the wall.

This sliver of light was all the encouragement I needed. I threw myself at the crack in the wall, clawing to let in just a little more light, a little more air so our relationship could breathe. "I thought a lot about it too," I said, revealing that this was of huge consequence to me as well. "Can I share my conflict with you?" I asked. "Part of me wants to recognize that, against all odds, you are pushing yourself to go to school, to do your work, to carry on even with a massive hole in your heart. Part of me feels that you are old enough to make your own decisions about whether now is the time that you want to be in therapy. At the end of the day, though, I am not ready to let you go. Our relationship is too important to me, and I think it might be important to you too."

And then I stopped talking, my intuition battling my insecurity. Emotionally exhausted, I leaned against my side of the wall and waited for a response that my ears would never hear. This time, though, I felt a different kind of silence in the air. I felt a silence that two might share when they are in each other's presence, together considering an all-consuming task. As I quieted my own sirens of self-doubt, I could feel the closeness between us. It was a hidden gem, smothered in Mandy's dread of abandonment, but it was there.

The next session began like many others, with a long, uninterrupted silence. About ten minutes in, Mandy looked up at me and said, "Okay."

"Great," I countered and then, "Okay what?"

"I'll keep coming. But once I go to college, that's it," she said, holding my gaze.

"Deal!" I shot back, trying to minimize the emotion in my voice. I wanted to recognize how hard it was for her to reach out to me in this way, but again, my gut told me to express it without words.

I spent the next few sessions stoking the embers of connection that our mutual fear of losing each other seemed to ignite. I began to allow myself to relax more with Mandy and with the wall she kept between us. With this acceptance came a more nuanced understanding of the meaning that this border held for both of us. I knew that the wall helped her manage the threat of closeness and her fear of rejection. I also realized that while the border kept me at a distance, it acted as a magnet as well. The border drew me close. I listened more carefully for possible invitations and scanned more vigilantly for signs of the slightest break in the wall. Each session felt like a personal challenge to make contact, to be smarter and somehow understand better what Mandy felt and needed despite the lack of clues. I wondered if Mandy believed that it was her wall, not her, that made me care so much and try so hard. I wondered if she feared that I would lose interest should she ever stop working so hard to maintain this barrier between us.

For me, the safety of my consulting room was one of the few places that I didn't summon a tall, firm wall of my own. Though I tend to be a private person and am not quick to share my feelings, I am arguably my most emotionally available with my patients. As such, Mandy's high, impenetrable wall both struck a chord and hit a nerve in me. I, too, am allergic to feelings of rejection, and I understood Mandy's need to protect herself. At the same time, her wall felt rejecting to me, and this was hard to manage week after week. Despite my own waves of discomfort, I was committed to staying with Mandy, bearing the wordless sessions and grappling with my own feelings of futility, loneliness, and hurt.

I began to appreciate more deeply Mandy's willingness to just be in the room with me and tolerate what must have felt like my endless stream of questions. I understood just how difficult the act of simply being with another was for her, as this "being together" ignited the near-constant duel within her between longing and her fear. As I allowed myself to relax more with Mandy, I stopped prioritizing the production of words between us. I think Mandy felt this shift in me, and as she felt more accepted, she too seemed to relax more in sessions. I finally realized that Mandy would not be fixed with words. It was the connection between us and what I could offer her in our relationship that would lessen Mandy's loneliness and sadness and bolster her self-esteem and very fragile self.

I marveled at Mandy's extraordinary courage as she silently battled her decade-long depression, the loss of her father, and the pressures of high school. During her junior year, Mandy was able to invest a little more energy in her schoolwork. She took an introductory class in law and, much to my surprise, decided that she wanted to be a lawyer. "Not a lawyer like my mom," she clarified. "A lawyer who does something that matters – like fight for endangered species of birds and the environment."

"I can't think of a more meaningful, more Mandy-like thing to do," I offered as I struggled to hold back the tears of relief and pride that I was feeling.

The second semester of her junior year fast became a time of increased activity. There were SATs, driving lessons, and, eventually, college applications. She still hid in her room and had little interest in anything that smacked of typical adolescence, but Mandy was moving forward. How she would handle dorm life, a roommate, and the social and academic pressures of college was anyone's guess. But I was committed to accompanying her on her near-wordless journey for as long as she needed me. I would keep the unspoken promise that I had made to Mandy and her parents three long years before.

If I Could Turn Back Time

Looking back, I wonder if my treatment with Mandy was successful. Even today, in my quietest moments, I am still unsure. Mandy has moved forward with her life and, as far as I know, has not succumbed to a deeper depression. In my last contact with her, I learned that she was finishing college and was preparing to apply to law school. My uncertainty reflects my personal style of pushing hard for what I want – acceptance has always been a much more challenging road for me. Rather than signaling an empathic choice to meet Mandy where she was, acceptance in my work with her felt like my fallback, made necessary by my inability to find a way past her protective walls.

Thinking about what I would do differently in this treatment, with analytic training and a decade more of experience behind me, several answers are clear. If I could turn back time, I would understand Mandy's silence and how I should work with her differently. In keeping with Macintosh's (2017) analysis of her work with a silent and self-destructive adolescent, I would understand that Mandy's silence held her despair and isolation. Her silence filled the treatment room with these feelings so that I could experience her most desperate emotional experiences.

Mandy's silence facilitated her emotional regulation, enabling her to tolerate her overwhelming sadness and continue to split off her anger. It offered her a sense of control over her longing for and dread of closeness with me, including her fear of betraying her mother by forming a close relationship with me. Speaking only minimally with me was her compromise – her way of being with me while not fully being with me. Far different than the classical view of silence as resistance, silence was Mandy's best attempt to communicate and share her inner world with me in the only way that felt bearable to her.

If I could turn back time, I would stop pushing Mandy to respond to me with words. I would heed Grossmark's recommendation, "Listen to your patient and be the analyst that your patient needs you to be" (2018, p. 24). I would tune in more to the messages she silently but poignantly communicated through her unique way of being with me. So many of our patients deluge us with spoken words to connect with us, to help us understand them, and, sometimes, to ensure that we don't understand them. Mandy rarely spoke but communicated the emptiness and loneliness of her inner world with an immediacy that for some time, I failed to grasp. The long, painful silences that we shared, the hopeful glances in which she would briefly catch my gaze, the occasional twitching of her pursed lips, or the child-like kicking together of her sneakers were all powerful communications. Today I would hear her silent communications and celebrate her willingness to simply be with me and risk the feelings of closeness that eventually emerged between us.

In hindsight, I see much of our work together through the lens of a long enactment in which Mandy invited me to share the emptiness, despair, and isolation of her internal world. As I sat uncomfortably in long wordless sessions, old experiences of isolation were triggered. I sometimes imagined we were prisoners, enveloped by darkness in adjacent cells, in the bowels of a medieval castle. When she spoke, a beam of light would barely illuminate our barren surroundings, and for that glorious moment, I felt I was not alone.

Today, I also have a deeper understanding of the enacted dance that Mandy and I were doing throughout our work together and the role of her silence in that dance. Over and over, I tried to cajole Mandy into speaking my language of audible words, consciously driven by my wish to "help" her and my certainty that I could best do so by helping her put her feelings into words.

In addition, I realize that Mandy's silence reminded me of past painful feelings of exclusion in my own family growing up and of my mother's occasional but deadly use of "the silent treatment" when she was angry with me.

For Mandy's part, my pressuring her to talk and her refusal to do so was a repetition of her relationship with her mother. In their relationship, Mandy's needs were secondary to her mother's needs for Mandy to feel better, function better, and to make her feel like a good and competent mother. In this light, I now understand Mandy's reliance on silence as a vital tool of self-assertion and a means of protecting her emotional experience from the judgments, intrusions, and criticism of important others.

If I could turn back time, I would have more faith in the power and meaningfulness of my connection with Mandy. I would value my being with her, in the way she would allow me to be with her, through years filled with loss and sorrow. I would consciously utilize Grossmark's (2018) concept of companioning and his urging that the therapist join the nonverbal patient in their dark and lonely internal world. Today, I see this as an extension of Kohut's empathic immersion. If my patient was unable to tell me about her experience, I would immerse myself in her nonverbal world. I would see, hear, and feel her communication, and I would tune in to the thoughts, feelings, and even physical sensations that I experienced in her presence.

If I was working with Mandy today, I would dive into the wordless work that my gut was telling me to do, and I would better manage my own feelings of self-doubt. I would find solace, if not pride, in communicating with Mandy within her register. This focus on Mandy's implicit communication might have allowed her nascent self to emerge more, without fear that it would be examined and critiqued.

Finally, if I could turn back time, I would still choose to get Mandy a birth-day present. While this gift was the acting out of my wish to "mother" Mandy and brighten her emotional world, it was also part of a "generative enact-ment" (Atlas & Aron, 2015) in which I longed to reach Mandy's potential self. In the precious moments of gift giving and gift receiving, I believe that I succeeded in this. This "moment of meeting" (The Boston Change Process Study Group, 2010) led to a session filled with dialogue, laughter, and the unmistakable experience of closeness. While my hope that this visible experi-ence of emotional connection could be sustained was unrealistic, it was still a lived experience between us that I believe was deeply meaningful for Mandy. I know it was for me.

References

Aron, L., & Atlas, G. (2015). Generative enactment: Memories from the future. *Psycho-analytic Dialogues*, 25(3): 309–324.

The Boston Change Process Study Group. (2010). *Change in psychotherapy. A unify-ing paradigm*. W.W. Norton and Company.

Grossmark, R. (2018). *The unobtrusive analyst: Explorations in psychoanalytic com-panioning*. Routledge.

Macintosh, H. (2017). A bridge across silent trauma: Enactment, art, and emergence in the treatment of a traumatized adolescent. *Psychoanalytic Dialogues*, 27: 433–453.

7   The Heartbreak Kid

Introduction

I recall as if it were yesterday, being seventeen and overwhelmed with the need to turn down the volume of my raging emotions. I can still feel the burn of an anger I wasn't able to put into words and the desperate need to define myself as different in every way from my parents and siblings. And I can remember how I used drugs and alcohol as a magical solution for these uncomfortable emotions – a solution that eventually demanded a very high price. Though I was able to make different choices than Jamie at important crossroads in my life, I could feel the pulse of her conflicts, and I understood the forces behind the damaging decisions that she made.

The next story, "The Heartbreak Kid," is Jamie's story. Whereas my self-destructive side had occasionally grabbed the steering wheel earlier in my life, Jamie's self-destructiveness was firmly ensconced in the driver's seat and had been making most of the decisions in her life since mid-adolescence. This is the story of her struggle with debilitating feelings of anxiety, inadequacy, and self-hate. It is also the story of Jamie's battle with addiction and our four tumultuous years of work together.

The Heartbreak Kid

It was a cool Monday morning in early spring when the quiet of my office was shattered by a shriek. As I pressed the message button on my phone, I was accosted by a woman's frenzied voice. "Hello. Hello . . . Dr. Feldman? Is this Dr. Feldman's office? This is an emergency. My daughter is being released from a detox and definitely can't go back to college. She's a disaster right now, a complete disaster. She needs a therapist immediately, and you came highly recommended. Can you see her? When can you see her?"

I glared at my phone as this distraught mother's voice reverberated with a raw anxiety that cut through my early-morning calm and made my stomach tighten.

Though I have received many similar phone calls from terrified parents and furious spouses, I was momentarily flustered by this mother's panic.

DOI: 10.4324/9781003543343-8

I wondered just what kind of disaster this young woman was – a raging bull ready to rip a well-meaning therapist to shreds or a delicate flower, losing vital parts of herself with each strong breeze? I was interested in finding out but needed to finish my first cup of coffee before I got this very overwhelmed mother on the phone.

Jamie was a twenty-year-old college dropout when she began treatment with me. Her mother told her that she needed to begin therapy if she wanted to continue living in their home, and Jamie knew better than to argue when her mother's anxiety was on fire. In her mother's eyes, Jamie had gone from being an attractive high school girl with mediocre grades and an outstanding musical ability to the emaciated and self-destructive drug addict whom I met after she failed out of her second year at a state university. While there were struggles within Jamie that her mother didn't notice as she grew up, she now clearly understood that her daughter was in the middle of a dangerous downward spiral.

The treatment promised heartache from the very first session. Jamie was a petite young woman with long, light-brown hair that looked like it hadn't been brushed in days. She wore skinny jeans, a baggy tee shirt, and old, dirty sneakers. Jamie had a disorganized and disheveled presentation, as if she had overslept for our 4 p.m. consultation and was still in the process of waking up. In short, Jamie was a train wreck, yet I liked her immediately. She led with a sweet, people-pleasing demeanor that was sprinkled with touches of sarcasm. Underneath this façade, Jamie was lying, stealing, and using pills, alcohol, and pot daily. Despite her superficial pleasantness, I sensed a simmering rage in Jamie and a keen intelligence, both of which were struggling to break through her narcotic haze.

Jamie strolled into the room for our first session, examining my office but avoiding the eye contact necessary to examine me. She sat in the farthest seat from me and opened with a casual "Hey."

"Hey," I responded and after a brief pause, added, "So, what brings you here?"

"Well, I don't want my mom to have a heart attack, so I thought I better show up," she half joked.

"Good call," I quipped, and after about thirty seconds of silence, I added, "She may have arranged the session, but it's yours now. What would you like to do with it?"

Without missing a beat, Jamie looked up and responded, "I'm anxious, I'm depressed, and I do too many fucking drugs. Oh, and my mother's making my therapy appointments."

Game on, I thought, silently admiring the wit and humor that were proving to be a welcome surprise.

I quickly learned that Jamie grew up the younger of two girls and had a pleasant but distant relationship with her sister, Dana, who was five years her senior. Dana was the perfect child. She was smart, popular, and well-behaved, whereas Jamie was the scatterbrained girl who couldn't sit still.

Bridget, Jamie's mother, was a secretary in their pediatrician's office, and her dad, Frank, was a consultant who traveled three weeks out of every month. Her parents had divorced when Jamie was four, but the two maintained a cordial relationship throughout Jamie's life. Bridget was the on-site disciplinarian and struggled for control over every detail of her daughters' lives. Frank was the unavailable father whose love and approval both girls desperately craved but rarely received.

As Jamie told the story of her childhood, she painted a picture of a lonely girl who was more than a bit out of step with her peers. Sweet and quirky, musical but not attuned to the melody of social interactions, she had had only a few equally awkward friends as a child. Jamie struggled with reading and found it nearly impossible to sit still through the endless school day. Her mother couldn't understand why Jamie didn't do better academically and complained constantly that she was lazy and unpopular with her peers. Bridget anxiously barraged Jamie with suggestions about how she could be more like her older sister.

Jamie grew up feeling overwhelmed and struggled to meet the normal demands of everyday life. Perhaps she was lazy, as her mother insisted. She certainly believed she wasn't smart enough or pretty enough to be successful in her parents' world. She saw her peers as more appealing and more capable but also as self-serving, untrustworthy, and ultimately, rejecting.

For Jamie, drinking and getting stoned every day in high school changed everything. When she was stoned, the anxious and insecure Jamie took a back seat to the seemingly carefree and indifferent Jamie. When she was drinking, the sad, lost little girl in Jamie often retreated as the defiant, self-destructive adolescent took center stage. Despite enjoying the relief that her new personas offered, the feelings of not fitting in persisted, and Jamie leaned hard on drugs and alcohol to soothe them.

Bridget loved Jamie fiercely and tried desperately to be a good mother. By the time I met Bridget, however, anxiety had transformed her into a chronically frantic woman. She was terrified about her lack of control over her daughter's behavior and became increasingly intrusive and overbearing with each crisis. Bridget insisted that Jamie call her every two hours and come home by midnight. Jamie ignored these edicts, just as she ignored her mother's demand that she wake her when she came home each night so that she could assess how badly Jamie was stumbling and slurring.

As I listened to Jamie's complaints about her "crazy, controlling mother," I felt the weight of the unappealing role I was about to be cast in – that of the anxious, overbearing therapist.

I knew that to optimally help Jamie, I would need to contain at least some of her mother's anxiety. Bridget needed to use me as a safe harbor to vent her panic and rage, and the three of us decided together that she could send me texts or leave voicemails on an as-needed basis. We agreed that Bridget could share information with me, but I would not violate Jamie's confidentiality and, therefore, would not answer most of her mother's questions. To her credit, Bridget understood this boundary, and despite her periods of overwhelming panic, she rarely pushed for answers that I couldn't provide.

While Bridget's anxiety was understandable, it was difficult for me to tolerate, even in very small doses. As a mother myself, I empathized with her fear for her daughter's safety and her worry and anger over Jamie's chronic dishonesty and reckless acting out. But Bridget's pressured speech, shrill voice, and overwhelming need for reassurance made me want to tune her out by whatever means necessary. I understood Jamie's drug use as one way to scream, "Stop!!!!!" to the mother who constantly harangued her and as her only way to quiet the version of her mother that lived in her head. I, too, wanted to scream when Bridget was revved up but settled for simply rushing her off the phone.

Despite her ongoing drug use, Jamie never missed a session during the first year of treatment. She was pleasant, compliant, and often insightful. In the early months of our work together, Jamie spoke about her wonderful but wonderfully dull ex-boyfriend, who she left behind during her senior year of high school when she graduated from weed and wine to pills and cocaine. Derek loved her and cried when he found her passed out in a friend's car with vomit on her pants and scrapes on her forehead and forearms from the evening's falls. The excitement of the drug deal and the dark glamour she found in snorting cocaine and taking prescription pills held a greater allure than Derek's quiet devotion. The anesthetic relief she found in drugs seemed to be the salve she had longed for as she struggled to manage her overwhelming anxiety and feelings of inadequacy, including her concerns about the demands of college.

As our work evolved, Jamie began to connect a lifetime of feeling like an "awkward kid" to her low self-esteem and crippling social anxiety. She came to view these emotions as the triggers for her drug use, along with her need to strike out against the overbearing mother who she loved, hated, and desperately needed. Jamie notably avoided talking about her shame at dropping out of college, her father's lack of interest in her, and her fear that hard drugs were taking over her life.

I felt encouraged by the close relationship Jamie and I were forming. I was surprised by her openness about her drug use and her ability to delve into painful feelings from childhood. Jamie seemed reassured by my ability to listen to the very disturbing details of her self-destructive behavior without becoming judgmental or panic-ridden or insisting she stop.

I told her when I was concerned about her and why, and I always emphasized my appreciation for her trusting me with the gritty details of her life. I didn't realize at the time how anxious Jamie was making me or, like her mother, how angry I was becoming in the face of my feelings of helplessness. Needing to manage my own discomfort, I shut down these feelings in favor of a more intellectual exploration with Jamie of the emotional triggers for her drug use and the risks and costs of her behavior.

After a year and a half of treatment, I received a flurry of frantic voicemails from Bridget. Jamie had stolen money from her and used it to purchase a large supply of pills. Bridget was worried that Jamie was not only using pills but dealing them as well. Over the next few days, a panic-stricken Bridget informed me that Jamie had not come home at night and was not returning her phone calls and texts. She begged me to contact her daughter and make sure she was all right.

I wrestled with this request. I wanted to avoid acting on Bridget's anxiety and doing her parental bidding, but this was unusual behavior even for Jamie, and I was quite concerned. I told Bridget that I didn't believe that calling Jamie, clearly at her mother's request, would benefit my working relationship with her daughter. I assured her that if Jamie didn't make our appointment in two days, I would reach out to her.

Much to my surprise, Jamie did show up for our next session, appearing foggier and more disheveled than usual. She drifted into my office with a sweet "good morning" and launched into, "My mother is so annoying. She is constantly telling me what to do and complaining about everything I'm not doing. Like leaving my sneakers in the foyer is a big fucking deal. She doesn't understand me, and she's always finding something to bitch about."

When she finally stopped ranting, I responded, "While that does sound annoying, I wonder if that's what we should be focusing on today."

After a brief silence, Jamie countered "I get it. My mother called you. I'm twenty-two fucking years old. I shouldn't have to check in with her every day. She just can't let go a little."

"She did call me. She was quite worried. How should she, or for that matter, how should I respond to what your mother told me – that you stole money from her and bought a large supply of pills?" I asked as matter-of-factly as possible. Her refusal to acknowledge the severity of her recent behavior and instead focus on her mother's imperfect parenting was making me angry. I was beginning to feel out of control in the treatment, as her addiction seemed impervious to my efforts and continued to spring up like a field of dangerous weeds.

As Jamie's antisocial and dangerous acting out increased, she buried her head deep in the sand to avoid looking at the risks she was taking and the people she was hurting. And Jamie was predictably more combative with me when I tried to get her to look at her dangerous behavior. The feeling that we were in a battle of wills should have been a signal that the angry parent in me was in the driver's seat and prompted me to back off and self-reflect.

Instead, my overwhelming feelings of frustration and helplessness impelled me to want to "do something" – an impulse that is never good to act on. I decided to take on Jamie's refusal to acknowledge how dangerous her behavior was becoming. I felt a pressing need to help her viscerally feel the toll that her drug use was taking on her and on those who cared about her. My grandiose plan was to finish by pointing out that this behavior seemed to be her way of silently screaming "fuck you" to the parents and therapist who, each in their own way, had not been able to understand her or meet her emotional needs.

"Listen, my friend," I started. "You are a mass of contradictions. How should we understand that you are a rock star in here and a complete mess out in the world?"

"I wouldn't say a complete mess," Jamie teased. "I think you are being dramatic."

"Maybe," I responded, "but this is exactly what I mean. You're funny and smart with me, but you are stealing from your mom and copping buckets of Percocet. I think you want to focus on this little shit with your mom and protect both of us from how bad things have really become. You don't want to look at how out of control your life is right now and what it's costing you."

Jamie was uncharacteristically quiet for a moment, and then, as her drug-abusing self-state reared its head, she looked defiantly at me and said, "I don't think so. My mom makes too big a deal of things, and you are too. I just like to get high sometimes."

"Sometimes?" I repeated, with more of an edge in my voice than I had intended. "How is that working for you?" I asked, my frustration clearly beginning to show.

I now felt her mother's urge to scream and ground Jamie for life. She was making light of her life-threatening behavior and was making me feel like an overreacting, middle-aged windbag who had forgotten how to have fun. I wanted to lay out the evidence on a table in front of Jamie, slam my fist down a few times, and drag an honest reaction out of her.

Instead, I finally caught myself and stopped talking. I allowed the silence, her anger, and my own frustration to fill the air. I felt like it was quiet for an hour. I knew that there was something going on between us that I didn't fully understand, and I wondered if part of me was punishing her with my silence. *Too bad*, I thought. *Nothing else was working*. With that, I understood just how inept and angry I was feeling.

I realized that Jamie and I were enacting what had happened between Jamie and her mother throughout her life. Bridget's anxious, intrusive responses to Jamie's social and academic challenges as a child left her feeling helpless, defective, and angry. As a teenager, Jamie began to use drugs to quell these and other unprocessed feelings. Her self-destructive behavior induced feelings of helplessness and anger in Bridget and in other adults who tried to control her. Jamie was inducing these unbearable feelings in me and, not surprisingly, I was feeling like I could use a drink. Worse than that, I was beginning to behave like an anxious, angry mother. It was time to get honest with myself and with Jamie.

I sat in session, silently wrestling with my own anger. Finally, I tried to describe what I thought was happening between us. "I think what's happening here is very much like what happens between you and your mom. You're in pain and don't feel like you can put it into words. Maybe you feel like both your mother and I couldn't handle your feelings if you did tell us about them. Your drug use is your way of doing something to quiet your overwhelming feelings. But then your mom gets crazy anxious and tries to control your behavior with anger and threats. And you defeat her with a giant 'Fuck you' by continuing to get high, which hurts both of you in the process. Does that sound about right?" I asked.

"So, now you're acting like my mother and getting pissed off at me? Is that what you're saying?" Jamie asked.

"Pretty much," I responded. "I have to do better, and I will." I was trying to validate Jamie's experience by owning my part of what was going on between us. I was also attempting to fortify our bond while not overwhelming Jamie with my own experience. To that end, I sat back and fought my urge to keep talking.

Finally, Jamie looked up at me and brushed the hair from her eyes. In a soft tone, she said, "I get it."

During this phase of our work, I battled my own feelings of omnipotence. I struggled with my deep-seated belief that it was my responsibility to make Jamie stop using, even though I knew that this was not a job that I or any therapist could succeed at. I knew intellectually that there were limits to how much I could help her, especially in only forty-five minutes a week. I reminded myself to keep a check on my own feelings of helplessness and a careful eye on the bond between us.

My urge to control Jamie's behavior was sorely tested when she began spending all her time with Kevin. I soon learned that Kevin was a twenty-eight-year-old heroin addict who Jamie met during her initial stint in detox, a setting he chose to avoid jail after being arrested for aggravated assault. Kevin was a low-level dealer who slept on the couch of his childhood home and was now clinging to Jamie as his girlfriend du jour and a pawn in his small drug-dealing enterprise. Jamie showed me pictures of the couple at the beach, both hugging a large beachball. Kevin looked like a strung-out version of Brad Pitt, and Jamie looked exceptionally proud to be by his side.

Within a few months of hanging out with Kevin, Jamie was getting high day and night and was helping him deal drugs out of his mother's basement. She lost her job as a waitress and again stopped coming home at night or returning her mother's desperate phone calls and texts. Bridget was understandably in a full-blown panic.

As the brewing crisis escalated, an overwrought Bridget left me a 2 a.m. voicemail. "Dr. Feldman," she shrieked, "I just got a call from the police station. She and that dirtbag got arrested. I don't even know what for. I don't know what to do anymore. I can't afford a lawyer, but I can't let her just rot in a dirty cell. Dr. Feldman, I don't know what to do."

By the morning, a shaken and seemingly remorseful Jamie was bailed out of jail and returned home with her mother. Three days later, she was right on time for our session and right back to minimizing the self-destruction at play.

Jamie began the session by prattling on about what type of restaurant she might work in next and about Kevin's plans for the two of them. I felt myself growing frustrated as I realized that she had no intention of bringing up her recent arrest. I felt as if she were toying with me, forcing me to play the angry parent to her reckless adolescent. She was projecting into me her feelings of being out of control, and consequently, I experienced an intense pressure to save both Jamie and our work together. I knew the lecture that I was aching to deliver was part of the script that Jamie had unconsciously written for me, just as I knew how useless my words would be. I searched my head and my heart for something authentic and potentially meaningful to say about how she was affecting me and just how concerned I was.

What finally emerged was "What the fuck, Jamie! I care a lot about you, and I have to watch you treat yourself so badly. It's really painful."

Jamie looked down, and for the first time, I saw her eyes filling with tears.

Unsure whether this was a manipulation or genuine affect, I said more softly, "Tell me about getting arrested."

Saturday night had been a trifecta of trouble, she explained. She and Kevin were snorting heroin and then went to deliver pills to a few high school kids. Suddenly, flashing police lights and blaring sirens were chasing them, and Jamie was terrified. Kevin's response to the police car behind him was to press hard on the gas, and his out-of-control car hit two other cars before it careened into a tree. Jamie was sobbing and shaking as the police pulled her out of the badly damaged car. She and a very belligerent Kevin were hand-cuffed and brought to the local emergency room. They were charged with possession and intent to sell illegal substances, and Kevin was charged with driving while impaired.

I had hoped that Jamie's frightening experience would become a pivotal point in her life and in her treatment. I desperately wanted this to serve as a "rock bottom" to motivate Jamie to confront the severity of her drug addiction and question her relationship with Kevin. I thought the courts might make rehab and ongoing monitoring of her sobriety part of a plan for Jamie to avoid jail. Regardless, I couldn't imagine that even Jamie's potent system of denial could withstand this kind of pounding by the hammer of reality.

Bridget was equal parts furious and frightened and vowed that regardless of what the courts said, Jamie was going to rehab the next time she was dis-covered using drugs.

I wondered what all of this would mean in my work with Jamie. Would she be willing to take an honest look at her self-destructive plunge? Could she trust me now that the courts were involved? And what of Bridget's newly felt justification to monitor and micromanage every fiber of Jamie's life?

With Kevin in jail and awaiting a transfer to rehab, Jamie began attending NA meetings and secured a job in a gardening store. She began spending more time with her mother and even got together with a few friends from childhood. Jamie found a sponsor and talked a lot about sobriety as well as her feelings of inadequacy and her social anxiety. I applauded her developing ability to turn to me and the NA program with these painful feelings rather than anesthetize them with drugs and alcohol.

About six weeks into this new world, Jamie began our session by sharing, "I'm not sure what to do. Kevin wants me to visit him and bring some stuff into the rehab. I'm kind of afraid to get caught. It's probably illegal or something."

While I knew that the addict inside Jamie was still alive and well, I had naively reassured myself that she was beginning to invest in healthy, supportive relationships and was getting a great deal of self-esteem from her involvement in NA. My disappointment that Jamie continued to be so drawn to Kevin and their shared world of drugs and danger was palpable.

"I'm glad you're bringing this up," I offered once I felt more settled emotionally. "Let's play it out. How do you see it working?"

"Which part?" she asked, being concrete as a means of avoiding the realities of the situation and her fear that she might disappoint Kevin.

"All of it," I replied. "From smuggling drugs in there to his using them and how you might get in trouble." I felt my anger with Kevin and my frustration with Jamie starting to brew.

"Well, he'd probably sell them," she volunteered, as if this were a preferred option to his using them.

I sat quietly, looking at her intently.

Eventually, she described her plan of sewing several bottles of pills inside a stuffed bear and bringing it to him.

"What do you think would happen if you got caught sneaking the drugs in or later if Kevin got caught with them?" I couldn't help but ask.

"I knew you'd think it was a bad idea. I don't even know why I told you," Jamie snapped petulantly.

"I do," I responded. "I'm pretty sure a very smart part of you agrees with me and thinks it's the worst idea we've both heard all year. That part of you is just coming up against the part of you that is desperate for Kevin's approval and is terrified of losing him."

The silence that followed was not the kind of silence I had hoped for, one that reflected deep thought or an emotional struggle. Rather, it felt like the kind of silence that informed me that I had been dismissed and that Jamie had already made up her mind. Despite her frail frame and sweet demeanor, I felt like I was wrestling with a mountain lion as I took on the addict part of my young patient, and clearly, I was losing. I considered asking her to explore what it would be like to disappoint Kevin or whether she was afraid that he would break up with her. I thought about asking her to describe the pull she was feeling to again immerse herself in Kevin's world – the excitement, the relief, and the inevitable self-hate that buying, selling, and using drugs brought. All these questions felt too intellectual and destined to fall flat.

Finally, I chose to focus on our relationship and to simply share my feelings with her. "Can I tell you what I'm feeling?" I asked.

"Sure," she said. "I know you're kind of mad and think it's stupid. I know you want to talk me out of it."

I spoke softly and slowly as I said, "Jamie, I just feel incredibly helpless and sad. I guess I'm afraid that I'm losing you. In some ways, you make me feel so hopeful. You're going to meetings and working hard in here. You're doing well at your job and even hanging out with old friends. But you have a self-destructive part of you that only trusts drugs to help you get by, and I feel like I'm running out of time to help you avoid really screwing up your life."

There was a long silence and Jamie looked up at me several times like a young child might look up at her mother after breaking a special vase. "I'm sorry. I don't know what to do. I promise I will talk to you before I do anything. Can I call you if I need to?"

"Of course you can," I assured her. "I know how hard these choices are for you." With that, I felt the tendrils of hope tease my sad heart and skeptical mind – always the harbinger of pain and disappointment when working with substance abusers.

Jamie did not call me. She missed our next session and didn't return my subsequent texts or calls.

Feeling concerned, I reached out to her mother. I was told by an angry and distant Bridget that Jamie had been on a using spree, financed by her mother's stolen diamond necklace. She was discovered passed out in the parking lot of a nearby supermarket three nights ago and was rushed to the hospital. Once she was well enough to be discharged, Bridget had dragged Jamie to a Salvation Army rehab several hours upstate.

Before I could ask any questions, Bridget stated flatly, "Thank you for your help, Dr. Feldman. Jamie is finished with therapy. She's just too far gone."

I quickly tried to quiet and compartmentalize my dueling feelings of worry and failure. I told Bridget that I understood her anger and disappointment. I suggested that we take things one step at a time and agreed that rehab was the perfect first step. Finally, I asked Bridget to have Jamie call me when she was able and to please keep me posted as to her progress and plans.

Despite my texts to both Jamie and her mother over the next several months, that was the last contact I had with either of them.

Losing my relationship with Jamie in this manner was extremely upsetting. Feelings of anger and frustration took a back seat to a more overwhelming experience of sadness and failure. I knew that working with substance abuse patients was always a roller coaster ride and that simply keeping her engaged in treatment for four years had been a challenge and an accomplishment. Still, I couldn't shake the feeling that helping Jamie had been within my reach, and I had somehow allowed her to slip away. Without an opportunity for closure, I was left to marinate in my own feelings of futility.

Fast-forward three years and I am getting lunch in a busy deli one town away from my office. I was certain that the young woman behind the counter wasn't Jamie, but she looked like a sober, healthier version of her. I remembered her emaciated frame, ragged appearance, and foggy brain. I reminded myself that Jamie might be dead or well into a lengthy prison term, given how badly her drug use had been spiraling out of control when our work together abruptly ended.

The very attractive, full-faced cashier glanced up at me, smiled broadly, and practically screamed, "OH MY GOD, Dr. Feldman! How are you? Do you remember me?"

The deli wasn't crowded, and Jamie was eager to tell me that three rehabs later, she was sober and had been for the past eighteen months. As she recounted her story of early recovery, I understood that the holding environment of a six-month inpatient program offered her the time and space to discover, rather than be told, who she was and who she wanted to be. During this time, it seemed that she found a kind of emotional understanding and protection that she needed to give voice to her rage, accept her anxious nature, and feel true empathy for the quirky little girl who lived inside her, the one who always felt that she didn't measure up.

As I listened to her story of bravery and hope, I felt those old twinges of frustration. I always knew that our weekly forty-five-minute sessions were no match for the enlivenment and escape that drugs offered. I had often shared my regret with Jamie that she refused more frequent sessions and only sporadically agreed to attend twelve-step meetings as an adjunct to therapy. I consoled myself with the belief that our relationship helped Jamie stay alive and tethered to the world of adults who cared about her until a more profound change became possible. As both witness and guide in my work with her, I had previewed with Jamie a saner path forward, toward a life that I wanted for her. I just couldn't convince her to leave drugs behind and walk that path with me.

I stared at this familiar yet unfamiliar young woman in amazement as she told me about the wonderful boyfriend she was living with and her full-time job. Her eyes seemed to sparkle. "I'm okay now. I've made it through the storm."

I wondered silently if she blamed me for not helping her enough.

As if she could read my mind, Jamie said "You hung in there with me when I was really awful. I always knew how much you cared. That meant more than you know!"

Her words were a welcome surprise. Later, I replayed our encounter in my mind. I saw her face, radiating health and resilience, and I noted the feeling that an old weight had been lifted. I thought that perhaps just being with her, not giving up on her, and staying as close to the heartbeat of her struggle as she would allow, was the best that I could offer at the time. Maybe, I considered, this was even enough.

If I Could Turn Back Time

My years of work with Jamie were filled with the kinds of soaring highs and plummeting lows that the treatment of young substance abusers often involves. Her limitless potential and sassy demeanor captured my heart, while her hair-raising penchant for self-destructive acting out caused me much nail-biting and more than a few gray hairs. Despite her impulsivity and difficulty with trust, Jamie remained emotionally connected to me through four turbulent years of treatment. Over time, she became increasingly able to turn to me rather than to drugs to help her regulate her intense emotions and manage her anxiety. But it simply wasn't enough.

If I could turn back time, I would encourage Jamie to bring her drug-addict self-state into our sessions more often. Relating directly with this part of her would likely have made her unmet relational needs, particularly those that were intricately related to her reliance on substances, available for conscious exploration (Director, 2002). For example, Jamie longed for an idealizable, calm, protective mother who could model how to manage her disruptive emotional experiences. In the absence of this kind of figure in her life, Jamie relied on drugs to feel powerful rather than helpless and to cope with her overwhelming needs, insecurities, and anxiety.

Inviting the drug-abusing version of Jamie into our sessions would have allowed her to see that I welcomed all sides of her and was prepared to go to the difficult and even unsavory places in which she dwelt. This would have been a crucial step in helping Jamie "stand in the spaces" (Bromberg, 1998) between the disparate versions of herself and would have reduced her need to dissociate the intensely painful affects that left her feeling alone and out of control.

If I could turn back time, I would focus more with Jamie on the adaptive purposes of her substance abuse and self-destructive behavior in the hopes of increasing her insight and decreasing her feelings of shame. Growing up, her mother turned a blind eye to Jamie's emotional and social struggles as well as the learning difficulties that were doubtlessly related to her undiagnosed ADHD. Rather than help her manage these painful experiences, Bridget's anxiety exacerbated them, especially Jamie's feelings of defectiveness. One adaptive purpose of Jamie's drug use was that it offered her a predictable and reliable way to quell these debilitating feelings. Drugs never failed to accomplish this important job and did so in a predictable and timely manner. They also offered Jamie an identity through which she felt successful and a social group that accepted and celebrated her.

The adaptive function of Jamie's flagrantly self-destructive behavior involved its function as an emotional X-ray of her feelings of worthlessness and self-hate. With her alarming behavior, Jamie put these toxic feelings on display in a last-ditch attempt to help others understand the depth of her pain. Her acting out was a communication that even her mother finally heard – an undeniable plea that her world was spinning out of control, and she desperately needed help.

If I could turn back time, I would decode her behavior in this way and relentlessly offer our relationship and the twelve-step program to meet the emotional needs that she was relying on drugs to manage. I would not simply ask, "Did you think about calling me or your sponsor before you got high?" I would follow up by inquiring what she imagined it would have been like to reach out to me and what it would have taken for her to do so. I would role-play her calling me and her sponsor and talk through any concerns she might have had about how we would respond. I would bring her fear of rejection and feelings of shame to the forefront and understand with Jamie how these internal bullies relentlessly led her to use drugs and avoid help.

While I spoke with Jamie about how sad and concerned her self-destructiveness made me feel, I did not discuss my own anger or my understanding that drugs were Jamie's best means to vacate the rage that boiled inside of her.

"Fuck you! I am exactly what you made me!" her drug-abusing behavior screamed at her parents and at me. She had found the perfect way to make her mother feel the inadequacy and rage that she had felt as a child when her mother constantly criticized her and her father ignored her. And she vented her rage by forcing me to be a Greek chorus of one, standing on the sidelines while helplessly, and at times angrily, narrating the tragedy that Jamie was consciously and unconsciously playing out.

If I had it to do over again, I would focus more on how disconfirming her father's minimal involvement in her life was for Jamie – even more, perhaps, than her mother's chronic anxiety and criticism. Both Jamie and I colluded in focusing solely on the effect of Bridget's intrusive and critical behavior. Unearthing buried feelings of rejection, shame, disappointment, and anger related to her father's lack of interest in her would have been important. In hindsight, I think his seeming lack of concern about Jamie's drug abuse and his perfunctory phone calls and visits on holidays left both of us feeling powerless and unimportant – emotional experiences that were already overwhelming the treatment room.

Finally, if I could turn back time, I would have spoken more with Jamie about my feelings of helplessness and the real limits of my ability to assist her in her battle with addiction. Like many who gravitate toward substance abuse, Jamie's chronic feelings of helplessness as a child contributed to her reliance on drugs for a sense of omnipotent control over her internal state and over others in her relational world (Director, 2005, Dodes, 1990, 1995, 1996). Had I been more transparent about the feelings of helplessness that I experienced with Jamie, I could have modeled for her how to tolerate and manage this destabilizing experience with a combination of communication, limit/boundary setting, and acceptance.

To model managing my feelings of helplessness in a healthy way, I would have needed to be aware of my own struggle with omnipotence and acceptance. As I look at my clinical work through the lens of "If I could turn back time," I see a multitude of examples of my certainty that if I could just find the right words, deliver them in exactly the right way and at the perfect time, I could convince my patients to change their self-defeating ways. The upside of this belief system is my pathological optimism and hopefulness. The downside is my own struggle to accept that there are limits to my influence, and there is much that I cannot control.

References

Bromberg, P. (1998). *Standing in the spaces: Essays on clinical process, trauma, and dissociation*. The Analytic Press.

Director, L. (2002). The value of relational psychoanalysis in the treatment of chronic drug and alcohol use. *Psychoanalytic Dialogues*, 12: 551–579.

Director, L. (2005). Encounters with omnipotence in the psychoanalysis of substance users. *Psychoanalytic Dialogues*, 15(4): 567–586.

Dodes, L.M. (1990). Addiction, helplessness, and narcissistic and narcissistic rage. *Psychoanalytic Quarterly*, 59: 398–419.
Dodes, L.M. (1995). Chapter 7: Psychic helplessness and the psychology of addiction. *The Psychology and Treatment of Addictive Behavior*, 79: 133–145.
Dodes, L.M. (1996). Compulsion and addiction. *Journal of the American Psychoanalytic Association*, 44: 815–835.

8 The Boy With the Beautiful Smile

Introduction

When my daughter was fifteen, she was prone to asking personal questions at seemingly random moments. "What were dad's other girlfriends like?" she asked when we were driving home from her tennis match several towns away.

"Did I ever tell you about Cindy? That's the woman your father should have married," I playfully responded. As she shook her head, I continued.

"Cindy was certainly pretty enough. She was tall and thin, with long light-brown hair that she wore in a ponytail. She didn't wear makeup, and her clothes were all different shades of neutral. Cindy was pleasant, low mainte-nance, and painfully vanilla." Cindy didn't love sex, but I chose not to throw that in when talking to my fifteen-year-old. "I think she eventually became a nurse. Oh, and Cindy was a cat person," I added.

As we pulled into our driveway, Molly looked at me and very nonchalantly asked, "Mom, is Cindy real?"

"No, sweetheart, she's not," I answered with a smile, feeling more under-stood than I had in quite a while. There was a synchronicity to our con-nection that went beyond our mother–daughter bond. We simply "got each other." Our minds worked in surprisingly similar ways. This unusual sense of emotional synchronicity, what Kohut referred to as a "twinship" selfobject experience (Kohut, 1984), resulted in a closeness and an extraordinary under-standing between us. It was this kind of feeling of closeness and synchronicity that I experienced in my relationship with Josh, a young man whom I have been treating since he was fifteen.

The next story, "The Boy With the Beautiful Smile," centers around my unique relationship with Josh, while also exploring the benefits and potential downside of closeness, synchronicity, and feeling understood in the therapeu-tic relationship. Fueled by our mutual obsession with dogs, Josh was excep-tionally open with me and never seemed to feel that I was misunderstanding or judging him. His ongoing feeling that I just "got him" was both a help and a hinderance in our work as we struggled together through his jungle of anxiety, depression, substance abuse, and anorexia.

DOI: 10.4324/9781003543343-9

This story focuses on the magic and the missteps that can occur when the therapist and the patient are too in sync with one another and the treatment seems to be going too well. While our closeness was surely a catalyst for change, it also led both of us to split off our anger and dissociate possible conflicts between us. Josh's difficulty accessing more uncomfortable feelings such as anger and disappointment and my unconscious resistance to engage with this side of him, adversely affected his ability to grow emotionally and contributed to his need to sabotage his own efforts.

The Boy With the Beautiful Smile

"My son is fifteen. He may have some issues with food. He may have some issues with his sexuality too," Josh's father informed me in our first meeting.

"He has the most beautiful smile. Everyone loves him," Josh's mother felt compelled to add. They were concerned by their son's request for therapy but held fast to the image that this charismatic boy steadfastly projected and suggested that our acquaintance would probably be a brief one. They were both struggling to minimize the extent of their son's pain.

Josh's father, a successful cardiologist, peppered me with questions. Where was I trained? What was my approach to working with teenagers? How many years of experience did I have? If Josh did have an eating disorder, what would my approach to this be? Josh's mom sat quietly, head down except for when she was studying the photos of my terriers, greyhounds, and poodle mixes, past and present, on my bookcase.

Toward the end of the consultation, I asked Josh's mom, "Do you have any questions?"

"Not one," she said with a soft confidence that surprised me. "You're a member of the tribe."

"The tribe," I repeated, assuming she meant that I was Jewish, as were they.

"You are a dog person. Josh will talk to you."

I met Josh when he was a sophomore in high school and immediately realized that his mother did not lie. Josh was warm, sweet, and truly had the most beautiful smile. Underneath the beautiful smile, however, he was in the throes of anorexia, pot addiction, concerns about coming out as gay, and struggles with anxiety and depression. I was left wondering how he was able to maintain such a seamless persona in the face of so much inner turmoil. I was also left questioning why he felt the need to maintain this dazzling front and what the emotional cost for him had been.

Josh walked into every session with an offering. "Love those boots! They are so perfect with your outfit." Or "Great jacket. That is so your color." These jewels were offered at a time when my own young-adult children routinely mocked my signature habit of wearing the brightest of colors, including my favorite turquoise cowboy boots that Josh had complimented. His gifts were laser focused on conveying his approval of my uniqueness, a skill that touched my heart and offered a glimpse of his natural talent for intuiting the needs of others should he continue to pursue his proclaimed goal of becoming a psychologist. Josh never ended a session without giving me a fun tidbit about what one of his Shih Tzus was up to and without asking about my canine crew. Our shared passion for dogs fueled the synchronicity of our relationship and Josh's growing feeling that we understood each other.

In the first few months of our work together, Josh was able to give me a detailed description of the hour-to-hour agony of his eating disorder and seemed relieved that this wretched way of living was finally emerging from the shadows. Josh's food restriction, his obsession with thinness, his need to count every calorie, and his preoccupation with his distorted body image were like a tape replaying over and over in his head. Coffee was all he would allow himself for breakfast. A little too much milk in it was unforgivable and needed to be punished by reducing the already meager calorie intake allowed for his next meal. Lunch, which he put off until he got home from school, was a small yogurt or a few cheese sticks, something packaged so he could be sure that it didn't exceed two hundred calories. Dinner was more challenging, as this was a meal typically eaten with concerned family eyes watching and assessing how much he was consuming. In Josh's mind, hunger was his friend and a sign that he was strong enough to withstand his flawed body's demand for food. At the beginning of our work together, anorexia had its tentacles in every crevice of Josh's mind and was consuming most of his waking thought.

As we got to know each other, Josh told me that he was bisexual and planned to fall in love with a person, regardless of their gender. Emboldened by the time and space that therapy offered to try on this new identity, Josh soon acknowledged that he always knew he was gay. He seemed confident that his parents would embrace his sexuality, but the reactions of his teachers, neighbors, and classmates worried him.

Though only fifteen, Josh was filled with worry about leaving home for college and imagined that his parents' marriage would fall apart if he was not there to stand guard. His only sibling, his older sister, was leaving for college in ten months and seemed blissfully without concern about their parents' relationship. But Josh was desperately worried.

Josh's schoolwork got only scraps of his attention, and close friends found him preoccupied and disengaged. Every conscious thought was consumed with either judging the calories he had taken in and the imagined extra inches around his thin waist or worrying about his parents. The only moments of rest came each night when he got stoned, and even those moments were followed by overwhelming feelings of guilt and self-hate.

Session after session, Josh spoke about his feelings of sadness, anxiety, and self-hate. We wondered together about his fear of disappointing his brilliant father and his feelings of responsibility for his gentle, sensitive mother. His feelings and fears had been neatly managed by his eating disorder and were now surfacing more as we challenged his anorexia. As the split between his sad and self-destructive self-state and his charming, extroverted self-state became more conscious, Josh was able to experience and wonder about these very different parts of himself.

By his senior year of high school, Josh's eating disorder had improved tremendously, but he was still plagued with periods of intense anxiety, stretches of very low mood, and a reliance on smoking pot to tolerate uncomfortable feelings. He continued to worry about whether his parents' marriage would survive his leaving home and believed that they wouldn't dare blow up his world while he was watching over them.

"I think they secretly hate each other. It just kills me. They argue all the time, and my mom always seems so upset. He's so critical and makes a stink when things aren't exactly the way he wants them. Like he's in the fucking operating room and she gave him the wrong kind of scalpel. Then she gets hurt and angry and starts slamming doors and banging things around the kitchen. She says she's okay, but I can see how much it hurts her. I feel like I need to be there for them, but I really don't want to be," Josh confided.

"Do you need to be there to keep your father from leaving or to take care of your mother?" I asked.

"Both," he replied. "I feel like I can't look away, or it will all fall apart."

"That's a huge job, an impossible job, in fact," I said and then added, "It's much easier to control everything you put in your mouth than your parents' marriage."

Josh began to give me his trademark smile but then stopped. I was struck by the sadness in his eyes. He exhaled and let the silence fill the air. We both knew that we had our work cut out for us if Josh was going to be able to leave home and thrive in college.

As the treatment continued during Josh's senior year of high school, I was smitten by his warmth and relentless hard work in sessions. Yet I failed to fully appreciate that he rarely experienced uncomfortable feelings in the room with me. While anger was discussed intellectually, I never felt its force, and Josh was always quick to reassure me that he was okay. Josh protected both of us and our relationship from the sharp edge of his rage, just as he had always protected his parents and his relationship with each of them.

In a way, I admired Josh's success in circumventing his anger. I have had the occasional tendency to throw things across the room throughout my life. In high school, it was my tennis racquet. In college, it was a typewriter (remember those?). As an adult, I have sent two or three chairs sailing across the room. With some patients, I offer an example of one of my angry outbursts as an attempt to normalize the experience and expression of rage. I usually start with, "We all lose it sometimes," and tell the story of when, provoked by my son flexing his new muscles of adolescent indifference, I threw a chair across the room and dented our new refrigerator.

With Josh, however, I never brought this up. I was too impressed with his intellectual understanding of what was bothering him and his newfound ability to put so many of his feelings into words. Anger, particularly the ugly anger that turns your face red and makes your nose run, seemed antithetical to Josh, his gentle manner, and his beautiful smile. It wasn't until much later in our work together that I realized that both he and I were unconsciously colluding to avoid his anger and the possible ruptures in our relationship that his anger might cause.

Josh was able to launch and make it to college on schedule. He and I planned to meet via Zoom while he was away and in person when he was home on break. Josh tried to tuck his worry about his parents into the farthest corner of his mind. He dove into the freedom of being a gay young man in an accepting social environment as well as the pot smoking that fast became a daily part of his college life. Not surprisingly, Josh put little effort into his studies and quickly felt overwhelmed by the academic challenges in front of him. The stress of his schoolwork, made worse by his trademark avoidance and escalating substance use, resulted in debilitating periods of anxiety and depression. There were days in which the most Josh could do was walk his beloved pair of emotional-support Shi Tzus before going back to bed. During his first semester, Josh came face to face with academic failure, and it became clear to him that neither his charm nor his natural intelligence would be enough to survive in college.

By the middle of his freshman year, Josh stopped attending classes, missed many of our sessions, and wasn't returning my texts or calls for weeks at a time. Eventually, he texted me that he was in a dark place, unable to approach his work, and was relying on getting stoned and sleeping to quiet the deafening tape of self-reproach that kept playing in his head.

I was concerned that Josh had internalized a sense of himself as a boy whose only strengths were his charisma and good looks. I worried that he doubted his intelligence and his ability to function competently outside the orbit of his family. Josh had stopped talking about his parents' marriage or his fear that he was about to be unmasked as the only "not smart" one in his family, but both clearly lurked in the shadows of the sessions attended and not attended. The therapist in me wanted to challenge Josh's menu of avoidant behaviors and share my fear that he was sabotaging his attempt at separation from his family and his foray into young adulthood. The anxious parent in me wanted to deluge Josh with questions, warnings, and a million practical suggestions.

When Josh finally showed up for a remote session, we talked about his difficulty getting out of bed, his mounting anxiety as he felt unable to concentrate on his schoolwork, and his avoidance of even going out with friends. After a brief stab at being empathic, I insisted, "Josh, you need to show up with me, especially when you feel crappy and don't look so pretty. That's when you need to show up the most."

"I know. I know you're right. I just don't want to talk to anyone when I feel that bad. Sometimes, I just don't have it in me," Josh quietly responded.

"Can you try to find it in you, no matter how badly you're feeling? If you can just show up, I'll help you with the rest," I pleaded, feeling and sounding more like a nagging parent than I had hoped.

Josh's uninspiring excuses left me feeling ineffectual and unimportant. While I was aware of feeling worried, it took me longer to realize that I was angry as well. It was an anger born of feeling dismissed and superfluous, the kind of anger that I might have shared with another patient but snuffed out with Josh in favor of offering relentless encouragement.

"You can do this, Josh," I insisted. "Avoiding everything with weed and sleeping has always been your go-to strategy. How is that working for you now?" I asked.

"Terribly, I know," he countered compliantly. "I just feel out of gas. I feel shut down, like it's hard to get anything done."

The painfully nurturing mother in me was in full gear, and I continued, "Just show up for our sessions. Let's start there. No more disappearing acts, okay?"

"I got it. I may not have much to say, but I'll show up. I promise," he reassured me in his soft way that suggested that he, too, believed in the power of what we could accomplish together.

Despite his promises, Josh continued to miss our sessions. Eventually, I became aware of my anger toward Josh for jeopardizing all that he had worked for, for shutting me out, and for making me feel helpless and unimportant to him. When we finally met, I told him that I was unsure of how I should have reacted during his weeks of darkened communication and that I got both concerned and angry as I sat waiting for him. "Maybe for the first time, you and I aren't connecting like we usually do. I think you are feeling alone and like you are falling fast. For my part, I'm feeling shut out and helpless and more than a little pissed off."

With the sharp smack of authenticity, Josh seemed to wake up and began to talk about how paralyzed he felt by the pressure of school and his fear of failure. Together, we understood his overwhelming worry that he was simply a beautiful shell, too fragile and unformed inside to endure any prolonged struggle. But we still didn't focus on our relationship and the role that I was playing in his acting out.

Sharing my anger with Josh seemed to kick open a door to uncomfortable feelings that we had both kept firmly shut. As we emerged from the enactment that was homogenizing our interactions, our mutual and unconscious avoidance of anger, a new ability for directness developed between us. Josh talked about his concern that his intellectual mediocrity would be exposed should he take up the challenge of his schoolwork in earnest. He spoke about his fear of his father's icy anger and how diminished and inadequate his father's disapproval had left him feeling in the past. And Josh voiced his fear of how hurtful he might become if he allowed his anger to come alive with either his mother or me.

I expressed my hope that he would try it out with me and my confidence that we would not only survive conflict, but our relationship would grow stronger with this new emotional freedom.

At the start of his sophomore year, Josh recommitted to putting a hold on the disappearing acts. He promised to show up with or without his smile; he might be sullen, angry, or profoundly disconnected, but he would show up. Josh was majoring in psychology and gingerly began to hope that he might have the cognitive hardware to earn his doctorate in this very competitive field.

I silently cheered and calmly voiced my certainty that he could go as far in psychology as he chose to go.

Josh's grades improved markedly during his sophomore year, and he decided to pursue his dream of going to college in New York City. He was not accepted to his first-choice school for the spring semester of his junior year but decided to enroll as a nonmatriculated student. Impressed with Josh's steely commitment, I shared with him that I felt a different kind of energy emanating from him, one that was infused with fortitude and determination.

Living at home and again meeting in person, Josh approached therapy like he was training for a marathon. We tackled the emotional issues that jeopardized his ability to separate from his parents, succeed in school, and pursue intimate relationships. I was concerned about his use of pot as an avoidant defense and asked about his reliance on it to cope with uncomfortable feelings and acute stressors in school. Josh acknowledged getting high every night after dinner, often by himself and in lieu of going out with friends. He described it as the only way he could turn off the tape of pressure and self-reproach that played endlessly in his head. While his dueling fears of failure and success were anesthetized by the pot, debilitating feelings of depression followed periods of prolonged use.

"Let's understand what you're hoping for when you get high and just what it is you're getting," I suggested.

"I'm looking to hit the pause button on this tape that keeps telling me that I should stay in my lane – that working super hard and being super smart is part of my father and sister's world, not mine. I'm the pretty one, I'm not the smart one. The tape stops when I get high, but then I feel like total shit, and eventually, a worse tape starts," he confided.

"And the worse tape. . . ?" I asked.

"That I'm gonna fuck this up, and everyone will know that I belong behind a counter at Saks, selling expensive eyeliner, not in a graduate program," he shot back.

"That's a crappy deal," I told him. "You're looking to pot to help you feel more in control and better about yourself, and you wind up feeling like more of a failure. Josh, you can be pretty and smart and live in whatever damn lane you please – as long as you're able to put in the work. How about you and I work on those tapes together?"

Josh and I talked extensively about how pot helped him regulate his anxiety and his self-esteem and, when necessary, not feel anything at all. He agreed that he had an allergy of sorts to daily pot use and that this was connected to his painful periods of depression. Josh decided to only get high on the weekends when he was going out with friends. Instead, he would increase his use of exercise and journaling to help manage his anxiety. He built a fall schedule around his interest in clinical psychology and enrolled in two particularly difficult courses, statistics and research methods. Josh was excited to start classes and take on the challenge of raising his GPA at this new and exciting venue.

I felt extremely proud of both of us for the relationship we had built and the hard work we were engaged in together. I looked forward to our sessions and was buoyed by a self-congratulatory belief that I was going to help Josh ride this wave of self-actualization right into a Ph.D. program. Imagine my surprise when, despite Josh's grit and determination, he froze in place just when he needed to be sprinting toward the finish line at the end of his first semester at his "dream school." In a self-destructive plunge, Josh stared blankly at a computer screen for three days and was unable to complete his final paper for his most important class.

"I can't make our session." Josh's text explained. "I'm overwhelmed with work. My final research paper is due Monday. It's fifty percent of my grade, and I'm not getting it done. I'm sort of just sitting here. I can't get myself to write a word."

"More reason you need to come in. You, my friend, are at a crossroads. We need to figure out why you are shutting down when things get difficult," I chirped.

Josh continued to balk at even a phone session but promised he would call me over the weekend with an update. It was 9 p.m. on Sunday when I received his text that his research paper was still unwritten. He had contacted the professor and was denied an extension. Josh was wrapped in despair that he was going to fail research methods and lamented that he simply didn't have what it took to become a psychologist. "How am I going to make it in grad school if I can't even get through college? I'll see you Wednesday," he texted. "It's too late now."

Josh and I were both experiencing a deep sense of failure. I wondered how we had unwittingly colluded to "not know" that this significant area of dysfunction was still squarely in the driver's seat of his life. I questioned why Josh didn't bring his struggle with schoolwork and procrastination into our sessions before he was in the eye of the storm, battered by a paralyzing anxiety and demoralized by feelings of failure. I also asked myself why I didn't catch a glimpse of this silent struggle, if only in the shadowy absence of any talk about how he was managing his schoolwork.

Josh texted me on the Monday prior to our next Wednesday session. "I didn't finish. My dad tried to help, but it didn't matter. I just couldn't do it. So I failed the class. I'll see you Wednesday. I just wanted you to know," he wrote.

"I'm sorry you had to go through this. We will figure it out. Hang in there," I responded. I was feeling helpless and concerned about how Josh was going to handle his overwhelming disappointment in himself and the sense of betrayal that I had failed him.

I worried that Josh would give up and embrace his fear that he was neither smart enough nor emotionally strong enough to succeed in a competitive academic field. I was afraid he would abandon his intellect and bury his feelings of anger and disappointment. I imagined Josh leaving college, working days at a trendy boutique in the city and getting high every night. Most of all, I imagined him sinking into a pool of deep sadness and seeking comfort in the safety of his carefully crafted, beautiful shell.

Josh entered my office Wednesday morning with an undefinable twinkle in his eye. "Well," he said, "that was really something. I fucked up but good. That was incredibly exhausting. I spoke to the professor, and he won't let me withdraw. I definitely failed the class. So here's what I'm doing . . ." Josh launched into a description of the steps he'd taken, including contacting the office of students with disabilities and meeting with his advisor to sign up for another semester as a nonmatriculated student.

As I looked at Josh, I was momentarily speechless and overwhelmed with a medley of relief, surprise, and admiration. I saw the strength and resilience that we had been laboring to cultivate. I saw Josh, at twenty-one, a young man with a new kind of beautiful smile, one that shimmered with self-acceptance and determination.

In the wake of Josh's failing his research methods class, I wondered how disappointed he was in me that I had colluded in not knowing and not seeing his mounting anxiety and unconscious need to undo his hard-won success. Giving voice to my concern, I asked, "Josh, how do you feel about the fact that I didn't see this crash coming?"

"What do you mean?" he quickly responded. "How were you supposed to see what I didn't bring into our sessions?"

"I think you are protecting me. I didn't check in on your huge issue with procrastination. I didn't notice that there was little mention of your schoolwork in the month leading up to the end of the semester," I countered.

"Shit, Beth. You didn't do it on purpose. Where are you going with this?" he asked nervously.

"We're in this together, and maybe I was a little bit asleep at the wheel. Maybe we should both feel some anger and disappointment in me," I responded.

"I don't think that's fair. I think it's way too much of a reach. It's on me to bring my problems into sessions. I'm the asshole if I avoid it," Josh countered.

I paused a moment and then told him, "I think it's on both of us to wrestle with what's said and what's not said. I wonder, though, if you feel with me like you feel with your mom. That I can't handle your disappointment or your anger and that our relationship can't handle it." The room got quiet, and after a moment, I added, "For the record, I welcome your telling me when I mess up and when and how I've disappointed you."

Privately, I wondered whether I was worried about Josh's readiness for the intensity of graduate school, as he was still in transition from distracted teenager to fiercely intuitive and articulate young adult. Or was I remembering my own unspoken doubts about whether I had the cognitive hardware to succeed in graduate school? When I finally earned my Ph.D., I asked my mother if she ever thought that I would become a psychologist. "I only hoped you would stay out of jail," she said. The sting of her words reminded me that, like Josh, I, too, had stepped outside of my assigned role in my family in search of fulfillment and success.

As our work together continued, Josh struggled for a deeper understanding of the unconscious forces that led to his self-sabotage in front of his computer. Rather than shrink away, Josh now had the fortitude to take control of the situation, own his fear and ambivalence, and double down on his efforts to succeed academically. Diving into his twin fears of failure and success, Josh and I realized how both fed into his unconscious need to remain the beautiful boy who was adored by his admiring parents. In his internal world, if Josh continued to disavow his sharp mind, he wouldn't pose a challenge to his smart, successful father and would continue to be the cherished little boy his mother could take care of. As a success, he risked threatening his father as a competitive force and emotionally abandoning his mother with his independence.

Josh and I are both working on allowing ourselves to experience dangerous feelings such as rage and dread together. As we move forward, I am less invested in being the idealized therapist, and he no longer needs to be the perfect patient. As Josh dares to trust me to embrace and survive his anger and disappointment, he is unlocking the freedom to deeply experience all the intense emotions that lie behind his beautiful smile.

If I Could Turn Back Time

If I could turn back time, I would still cultivate and celebrate the close bond and unique synchronicity that made my relationship with Josh special and transformative. Josh has become a confident, determined, and engaging young man who is in a rewarding long-term relationship and is steadily pursuing his goal of becoming a clinical psychologist. I believe that our work together has been an instrumental part of his emotional and interpersonal development over the past nine years.

If I could turn back time, however, I would show Josh and myself sooner that our relationship would be deepened rather than threatened by more readily talking about uncomfortable feelings such as anger and disappointment as he experienced them in our relationship. I would encourage him to call out my misattunements and missed opportunities and to share with me what these ruptures were like for him. Together, we could then repair our bond and delve deeper into the painful feelings and old wounds that may have been triggered. In the process, he, I, and our relationship could grow stronger.

By colluding with his tendency to either dissociate or consciously avoid feelings of anger and disappointment in our relationship, I deprived him of the opportunity to work through his fears about the destructiveness of his rage. Had Josh been able to rail at me for not seeing his academic spiral before it was too late, I could have survived his anger, validated his feelings, and celebrated his new ability to experience and express negative affect. This would have also helped absolve him from his felt mandate to be the "protector" in close relationships at the expense of his own authentic reactions.

In hindsight, I would realize much sooner that I was engaged in an *in-actment* of "not knowing" with Josh prior to his freezing for days in front of his computer. I would listen more actively for what he wasn't discussing in sessions and address his long-standing tendency to avoid all that made him anxious. I would focus on his need to protect me, as he does his mother, from the ongoing severity of his struggles. Similarly, I would explore his fear that if he disappoints either his father or me, he will lose our attention and admiration. In other words, I would take on the parental selfobject functions and disappointments and explore them more directly from within the treatment room.

For my part, I would appreciate that I had basked in Josh's idealization of me. I would realize that my reticence to give up the role of idealized therapist was tied to my own narcissism and resulted in my inability to see the signs of Josh's academic spiral. Had I acknowledged the depth of Josh's anxiety, difficulty tolerating painful affect, and self-destructive potential, I also would have had to recognize that our work together wasn't going as seamlessly as I thought it was.

Reference

Kohut, H. (1984). *How does analysis cure?* 2nd ed., A. Goldberg (ed.). University of Chicago Press.

9 On Being Human

Introduction

As therapists, we are sometimes tasked with working while our own hearts are breaking and our minds are overflowing with worry. Life events such as illness, divorce, or death of a loved one may cause searing pain for months or years to come. Such challenges raise questions about when a clinician should continue to work and what, if anything, they should share with their patients. If a therapist does choose to work while grieving, what are the pitfalls and areas of vulnerability that could be anticipated? And how does this kind of challenge to a therapist's ability to focus increase the likelihood of ruptures, enactments, and misattunements?

The next story, "On Being Human," tells the tale of my work with Lydia during the excruciating weeks surrounding my father's death from COVID-19 one year into the pandemic. During our work together, Lydia and I helped each other, first, to survive and eventually, to heal. For both of us, leaning into simply being human, like turning into a skid on an icy road, helped us to regain a sense of direction and control in our own lives.

On Being Human

I sat in session with one ear trained on the quiet pinging of my phone, waiting for news from the hospital about my ninety-four-year-old father's condition. It was one year into the pandemic, and my father lay dying from an awful virus that precluded my holding his hand during his final days. My eyes were focused intently on the computer screen in front of me, and my other ear was struggling to listen closely to my new patient.

Lydia was an attractive and stylishly dressed thirty-four-year-old woman. She was the mother of three-year-old Brianna and a successful dentist with her own practice. While her manner appeared strong and direct, her voice began to quiver within the first few moments of our first session. Lydia tearfully shared that she was seeking help because her husband had gotten physical with her. That's how she put it, "he got physical."

"He hit you?" I asked, trying to clarify what she was telling me.

DOI: 10.4324/9781003543343-10

Then, slowly, Lydia told me the story that she had come to therapy to tell.

"I guess. I guess you could say that, but it's not like he punched me. He gets so mad, and if I don't back down, he just loses it. It's been like that for years. This time, when he started screaming at me, I told him that Brianna and I would be better off without him. I said that if he didn't watch out, we were going to my parents' and leaving him. I never said that before. The fight started out so stupidly. He was mad that I didn't want to go with him to watch football at his parents' house. It always turns into dinner, and Brianna gets cranky, and then his father starts making his critical comments. She's only three, for Christ sakes! I said to just go by yourself. Then he started complaining that what he wants never matters and I never want to see his parents. And now he's screaming."

Lydia told the story in an almost mechanical way, without the sadness in her voice that her red and puffy eyes suggested she felt. She paused as if not telling the rest of the story would somehow erase it from having happened.

After a long silence, I quietly said, "Go on."

Lydia took a deep breath and reluctantly continued, "I finally said, 'Stop being such a baby. I said I'm not going, and I'm not. Unless you're not very bright, it's just not that hard to understand.' That's when he grabbed me and half pushed, half threw me into our dresser."

I allowed her story to fill the room and let its impact wash over both of us. Finally, she looked up at me, and our eyes locked. Trying to replace the outrage I was feeling with as much calm and warmth as I could muster, I responded soberly, "Sounds awful."

This was followed by another long silence. I could feel her internal battle between shame and anger, neither of which she was ready to share. My inner voice told me to go slowly, that if Lydia said too much about either emotion right now, she might feel too exposed to come back for a second session.

"Tell me more about you and Vincent," I eventually urged, trying to convince both of us that there would be no rush to judgement.

Lydia talked about meeting Vincent when she was in her second year of dental school. Vincent was the owner of the car dealership where she took her RAV4 for servicing, and he was magnetically drawn to her from the moment their eyes met. He was charismatic and charming and pursued her relentlessly. Growing up, Lydia never received the expensive Christmas presents that her friends did. She never went on tropical family vacations. Lydia longed to feel special, even spoiled with attention and admiration from her caring but reserved parents. When Vincent bought her beautiful jewelry and took her out for fancy dinners and exciting weekends away, she was swept off her feet. Six months into their relationship, Vincent presented her with a new Lexus convertible and the keys to his apartment. The deal was sealed.

Lydia talked about the change that came over Vincent several months after they were married. "Suddenly, he took everything like it was a slight, like I thought I was smarter than him. He was sweet and protective when I was pregnant and when Brianna was born, but the past year, it's gotten bad again. We still go out and we still have fun. He's still the life of the party with our friends – really, my friends, but they think he's great. The sex is even still good. I still find him incredibly attractive, but he gets mad so easily and becomes a bully so quickly," she explained.

"How do you understand his rage?" I asked.

Lydia considered this question and said, "His father is a real asshole, a real rich asshole who always made him feel like he wasn't good enough. Even though Vincent is very successful, his father criticizes him constantly. So now, he does it to me. I'm just afraid of where this is heading and of how he is going to be with Brianna when she's a little older."

"Are you concerned that he'll become physical again?" I finally asked, unwilling to let the session continue without at least suggesting my concern.

"No" she said, "We fight a lot, but he never raised a hand to me before. I could tell he felt badly because afterwards, he apologized and said that he felt like I was coming at him and he just needed to push me away. He knows that's ridiculous. I've never been violent with anyone, and I'm certainly not going to start with a man almost twice my size."

We weren't through our first session, and I was already flooded with conflict. On one hand, I was concerned about the escalation in Vincent's aggression as well as his long-standing pattern of mistreating his wife. I silently cautioned myself to tread lightly as I realized how angry I felt after listening to Lydia's account of Vincent's thin-skinned bullying.

On the other hand, I knew that she was not in my office to be told to leave her husband. It seemed that Lydia had come to therapy for guidance and for validation that she was entitled to an intimate relationship that was not dominated by her partner's insecurities or aggression. I believed she was also in my office to develop the emotional strength necessary to protect both her daughter and herself. As she spoke, I watched the cracks in her defensive wall deepen as her need to minimize the abusiveness of Vincent's behavior collided with her recognition that an unspoken line had already been crossed in their relationship.

In the next session, Lydia talked about Vincent's pressures at work and how this contributed to his stress and irritable mood. As she spoke, I was having trouble focusing and kept thinking that I heard the pinging of my cell phone. Was it the hospital calling about my father's condition or one of my siblings with yet another devastating update? I felt my heart break as I strained to listen closely to Lydia. I sensed her quiet rage while I envisioned my father slipping out of my grasp.

As Lydia spoke, I thought about how she was victimized by her husband's rage, a rage born of his own father's rage. This ignited memories of my father fuming at faceless others for seeing the world differently than he did. Suddenly, I was back at the dinner table as a young child, whispering with my mother as my far-left father and older brother and sister discussed the problems of the world – my father ranting about the inhumanity of the right. A few seconds later, my mind shifted, and I was at the dinner table as an adult, ref-ereeing between my father and my more conservative husband, voices raised while arguing policy, as if each were setting it for the world himself. My atten-tion was held captive by my father's anger, a storm so intimidating that I often missed his deep empathy for those less fortunate than he was. These memo-ries flew into my awareness – like errant pebbles hitting my windshield – sometimes chipping and sometimes shattering my emotional wall, as I tried to speed forward in forty-five-minute increments.

Over the next few sessions, Lydia spoke about convincing Vincent to enter couples therapy by appealing to his love for her and his genuine wish for a closer, less conflictual relationship. Rather than focusing on Vincent's anger, as Lydia had hoped, the marital therapist concluded the first session by talking about Vincent's need to feel that she had faith in him and that his feelings mat-tered to her. This only reinforced Lydia's sense that her needs were invisible and her fear that if this baby boy she had married wasn't properly stroked, he would rain down an angry hell on her and their young daughter. As Lydia described the therapist's suggestion that she offer him the recognition he so desperately craved, she took more deep breaths than usual, and her eyes failed to meet mine.

"It feels like you have to swallow a lot of your own anger to get that job done" I told her, and I bristled for her at the high price of securing peace in their home.

I struggled with my own growing disdain for Vincent's self-absorption and abusiveness along with my wish to help Lydia run for the proverbial hills dur-ing many of our sessions. Trying to conceal my strong feelings, I compensated by asking, "Is there a part of you that feels any of the admiration you seem obliged to offer up, perhaps a part that's separate from all of the anger?"

"Of course," she snapped and then added more softly, "There are things that I love about him when he isn't being such an asshole. It just gets washed away when he acts like a bully."

"Have you told him that?" I too quickly inquired. As my words slipped out, I immediately understood that my concrete focus on better communication was my clumsy effort to manage my own feelings of dislike for her husband.

"That's the worst thing about it," Lydia uttered quietly. "He thinks he's com-pletely justified. He said he wouldn't be so mean if I wasn't such a bitch."

"What does he say about putting his hands on you?" I asked, now clearly angry and unwilling to be complicit in her denial of how out of control things had gotten.

"He swore it would never happen again. I believe him, but I told him that his screaming wasn't okay either. He gets that I don't want Brianna to grow up like he grew up, with screaming and fighting. I don't want to keep living like this either. He's talking in our couple sessions about his dad a lot. I think that's going to be helpful," Lydia said, trying to sound more certain than I believed she felt.

I shuddered as I felt the particles of self-doubt and self-blame in Lydia's words explode as they hit the air. I remembered struggling with my own feelings of self-doubt as a child when I was faced with my father's frequent ire. I wondered silently if learning to stand my ground in the face of his combativeness was the birth of my own resilience. As I thought about my larger-than-life father, my mind envisioned him lying alone, barely conscious, in his hospital bed.

I was focused on keeping my dislike for Vincent out of the treatment room and helping Lydia access her own disavowed rage when I suddenly recognized her pattern of subtly attacking his greatest vulnerability. When our bond felt strong enough, I asked, "Can we look more closely at what goes on between you and Vincent when you argue?" Recognizing that I was wading into murky waters, I added, "Nothing you said or did justifies his getting physical with you, but what do you think your part is in this dance with your husband?"

"What do you mean?" a surprised Lydia asked. "I'm just defending myself."

"I noticed how good you were at pressing your husband's buttons. For example, when you were arguing with Vincent, you seemed to suggest that he 'wasn't very bright,' knowing how sensitive he is about not having finished college. Do you think that hit a nerve?" I asked.

Lydia paused and then offered, "I always saw him as such a bully. Maybe I didn't think what I said could actually hurt him."

"Maybe you were just so mad at him that you wanted to strike back. And I think that you knew exactly which button to push," I countered, hoping to make her more aware of just how angry she really was and her role in their escalating conflict.

Curious to hear more about her childhood, I said, "Tell me more about your parents and your family growing up."

Without missing a beat, Lydia responded, "My parents were great parents. The five of us got along really well. There wasn't a lot of fighting. My parents almost never got angry. They always seemed like best friends, and they always supported me and my brother and sister. When I was little, we . . ."

As Lydia relived chosen moments of her childhood with me, I struggled to stay present with her. Was it my own pain beckoning, or did the emotional monotony she described simply not compel my attention? As she spoke, I thought about the contrast between her milquetoast upbringing and Vincent's charisma and explosiveness. Might this be why Vincent's intensity was such a draw to her? I wondered if an utter lack of vitality had silently infected my patient's childhood.

Some seek a partner much like their difficult parent in hopes of fixing that parent in their mind and getting the love that eluded them in childhood. Others choose a partner who is decidedly different from their difficult parent, attempting to meet important unmet needs left over from childhood. Lydia chose a husband who seemed to offer her the intensity and adoration that she craved, a man whose emotional makeup, for better and for worse, was vastly different from that of both of her parents.

My thoughts lingered on my father and her father – on a father's impact on his daughter. Lydia reacted to her father's passivity by seeking out intensity and enlivenment, the underbelly of which was Vincent's extraordinary inse-curity and poorly controlled rage. Fortunately, because her father raised her with patience and understanding, Vincent's relentless anger did not feel familiar or deserved. As this conflict unfolded in our sessions, I struggled to help Lydia access the fighter within her, the feelings of self-worth and her own split-off rage that she needed to stand up to her husband's abusiveness. I also tried to make her aware of her habitual way of striking back at Vincent that only served to intensify his feelings of inadequacy and escalate their conflict.

When the hospital called to say that my father had died, I didn't allow myself the kind of cry that begged to roar through my body. Rather, I prepared myself to hold my mother's hand and tell her that her best friend of sixty-five years was gone. Two days later, we stood graveside in the frigid cold of Febru-ary, surrounded only by immediate family in this new pandemic-forced way of saying goodbye. This was not the kind of ending my father should have had, not the send-off he deserved.

When my turn to speak arrived, all the memories of his anger receded. I heard myself thanking him for teaching me to live life with relentless pas-sion. I remembered aloud how he adored my mother and the extraordinary pleasure he took in his work. I listened to my son's voice break as he remem-bered his grandfather on the yearly vacations of his childhood, burying can-nisters of change in the Florida sand and then taking him treasure hunting. I thought of the picture my daughter had sent me that morning, of herself with her grandfather, both dressed in feather boas and tiaras, playing in her five-year-old bedroom. As this day neared an end, I wondered if in memory, I met a sweeter side of him that I had been too afraid to fully embrace.

There was no shiva during the early months of COVID, no visits from con-soling friends or relatives. I went back to work the next day, still heavy with grief and overwhelmed with worry for my heartbroken mother. I dove into each remote session, looking for a place to direct my attention and a distrac-tion from my own sadness. I felt a pressing need to be of help after feeling so helpless during my father's illness. While a part of me was concerned that I was seeing patients too soon after losing my father, another part of me knew that between his loss and my mother's impending decline, this tumultuous chapter in my life was just beginning.

My frequent questions eventually coaxed Lydia to reflect on her upbring-ing, and she began to talk about old, barely registered feelings of hurt, disap-pointment, and even anger from her childhood. Her mother's passivity, her father's lack of emotion, her sister's self-absorption, and her brother's anxiety had all been noted but remained unanalyzed.

As Lydia became increasingly willing to remember and self-reflect, she also began to more deeply experience her feelings of hurt and anger at Vincent's bullying. We explored her pattern of swallowing her rage until she reached a breaking point and then impulsively striking back at his vulnerabilities. We talked about the steps in emotional regulation that were missing – i.e., allowing herself to experience and identify feelings and then find a way to communicate them to her husband.

Lydia soon began responding to Vincent's provocations by looking him in the eye and saying, "I don't want to do this right now," and walking away. Later, when they were both calmer, she would tell him how she felt and why. Predictably, sometimes, this went well, and sometimes, it didn't.

As Lydia shared her new assertive strategy in their couple sessions, they were able to work on what it was like for Vincent when she "declared the fight over" as he put it. The couple therapist was able to reword this as "the screaming part of the fight was done," and suggested that the disagreement could and should continue when they were both able to think and speak calmly. To facilitate this, Lydia and Vincent agreed upon a sentence to put a pause on their fighting that he felt less threatened by.

During this time, my work with Lydia focused on helping her see the different sides of the people in her life and, importantly, the different sides or "selves" within her. Lydia talked about the "demanding little girl" in her that she instinctively kept hidden from her parents, certain that this side of her would elicit their disapproval. Vincent had intuitively sensed this part of her and had set out to win this little girl's heart with his enlivening attention and lavish gifts. I considered diving deeper into Lydia's feelings of envy and the resentment that lived within this "demanding little girl," but I sensed that it would only provoke an intellectual retreat at this point in our work together. Instead, we focused on her developing self-assertion and her becoming a far different wife and mother than her mother was.

After several more sessions, Lydia strode into my office and was eager to tell me about the previous night's conversation with her husband. "I told him that we needed to sit down and talk. I poured us each a glass of wine and sat on the couch next to him. I said that I want better for Brianna. I told him that I want her to have a father with my father's patience and with Vincent's big heart. And I told him that I want more for all of us than what he had growing up. He started to cry and said that he does too. Then he was sobbing, telling me how sorry he was. I've never seen him cry before, and I was almost scared. I told him how much I love him but that I will leave him if he ever puts his hands on either of us again. I really mean it, and I think maybe he knows that," Lydia shared with a medley of strength and sadness in her voice. In her words, I heard the soft drumroll of change.

As I proudly told her, "You are really brave," I saw a sparkle in her eyes and a glimmer of the fighter that was emerging from within her.

Lydia left my office, and I was alone with my thoughts. My mind drifted back to growing up with my father. In the face of his volatility, I learned to stand my ground. My feisty nature, my penchant for pushing hard, and my relentlessness were all my responses to his intensity. As I struggled to accept his loss, part of me wished that he had been a softer man during my early years. Another part of me understood that he helped create the fire in me that is a cornerstone of who I am today. It was this resilience that I saw stirring in Lydia's eyes, and I knew that we were on the right track.

In the wake of my father's death, this work that I love became both stressor and savior. Continuing to work during this time meant managing a heavy heart, a weary and fragmented mind, and a lack of emotional energy that was new and unnerving to me. As my emotional resources were stretched thin from grief, I often found myself running back to the safety of my patients' problems. At times, I tried to lose myself in their stories, riding the waves of their shifting emotions with them. At other times, it felt nearly impossible to compartmentalize my own pain and focus on anyone else's experience. I knew that Lydia needed access to the strong woman in me, as an idealizable figure who could help her cultivate her own feelings of self-worth, strength, and courage. These feelings, however, felt in short supply for me, and I worried that in this way, I was failing her.

Yet there were some positive surprises during this difficult time. When the dull ache of loss left me feeling lost and alone, my relationship with patients such as Lydia helped me to feel more connected and reenergized my sense of identity and purpose. While I sometimes struggled to think analytically in sessions, my emotional register was functioning more like a sensitive tuning fork, amplifying the rawness of my patients' emotions.

In my work with Lydia, I ached more deeply with her as she described feeling criticized and demeaned by her husband. I burned more intensely with rage as I heard stories of her being bullied and manipulated in the service of Vincent's fragile ego. And I rejoiced with greater abandon as Lydia embraced her own feelings of worth, strength and anger, and courageously began to thrive.

If I Could Turn Back Time

If I could turn back time, I would still have chosen to work with Lydia during this very difficult time in my life. Despite my heavy heart and distracted mind, Lydia benefited tremendously from our ten months of work together. She became more aware of her own internal experience, including her ambivalent feelings toward important others in her life and her conflicting needs and fears. By recognizing the different sides of herself, Lydia became stronger emotionally and more able to embrace her anger and effectively stand up for herself. With my help and that of their marital therapist, she and Vincent managed to deescalate the conflict that threatened their family and find more meaningful ways to communicate with one another.

If I had it to do over again, I would still have gone back to work immediately following my father's death. Seeing patients during the final weeks of my father's life and immediately following his death was a decision based on my defensive style, the unique circumstances of the pandemic, and my heartfelt belief that I could continue to meet my patients' needs. Unlike the moving accounts of clinicians who endured personal tragedies in Barbara Gerson's compelling book, *The Therapist as a Person* (2001), the death of my ninety-four-year-old father was not tragic, nor was it shocking. While I was extremely sad and overwhelmed with worry and responsibility, I felt able to compartmentalize my pain, and I utilized my own therapy and peer supervision group to support me in my grief and guide me through the challenge of working during this painful time.

My decision not to take time off prior to and following my father's death was profoundly influenced by the bizarreness of the times. Because it was during one of the deadliest phases of the pandemic, I had to fight for special permission to visit my father when it was clear that it was time to say goodbye. My twenty-seven-year-old son insisted on accompanying me onto the intensive-care COVID unit, where we donned hospital gowns and multiple masks and were instructed to stay ten feet away from my father. While we longed to hold his hand, kiss his forehead, and breathe in his presence one final time, we stood at a distance. Louis and I took turns telling my father, his grandfather, how much we loved him and how terribly we would miss him. And we reassured him that it was okay for him to let go, that we would look after my mother.

Then there was a family-only graveside burial and an hour-long, remotely held shiva. Because my siblings had health issues and were concerned about contracting COVID, I was left to help my devastated mother survive her first days and weeks of widowhood. With no office or gym to go to and no friend's house to visit, I was in desperate need of the distraction and purpose that continuing to work offered me.

My defensive style involved avoiding the depth of my emotional pain by compartmentalizing my sadness and keeping my worried brain busy. To that end, I focused on the many tasks that needed to be accomplished and the pain of select others that didn't threaten to shred my heart. It was through immersion in my work that I regained a modicum of control over my emotional world and moments of reprieve from the intensity of my loss. The decision to work through this difficult time may have been selfish, but at the time, it felt like a matter of survival.

I chose not to tell my patients about my father's death. My sadness and worry made me feel far too vulnerable to speak about my loss in sessions. I realized that patients who knew me well might have implicitly experienced certain subtle shifts in me. Perhaps I was a bit slower to respond or was more measured with my smile and laughter. I might have looked sad or exhausted. I prepared myself to handle any questions that my patients might ask. Whether no one noticed a difference or those who did sensed my need for emotional privacy, no questions were ever asked.

If I could turn back time, I would better understand the effect of my own stress, anxiety, and sadness on the way I worked. Typically, I would either immerse myself in my patient's inner world or focus on the here-and-now of what was going on between my patient and me in the session. In the wake of my father's death, however, I longed for a more concrete target for my attention and therapeutic energy. As a result, I was more laser focused on the details of Lydia's story each week and less attuned to both the murkiness of her inner world or to my experience in the room with her.

This restricted focus did not result in any notable ruptures, but it did represent misattunement in the form of missed opportunities (Gardner, 2024). I only paid cursory attention to how Lydia handled conflict earlier in her life – i.e., with her siblings, her parents, friends, and past boyfriends. I also didn't pay sufficient attention to how she avoided conflict with me, especially when I made misattuned or mistimed comments about her husband's abusiveness.

Lydia idealized me as a strong maternal figure who could teach her how to manage her husband's aggression, gain better access to her own rage, and further develop her feelings of self-worth. She soaked in my approval as she shared stories about how she was asserting herself with Vincent. Despite these facets of our connection, I felt a lack of intensity and a subtle distance in our relationship that I chose not to explore. If I had it to do over again, I would summon the intellectual and emotional energy necessary to analyze both my and Lydia's role in the distance between us. Perhaps I was simply too depleted to push for a deeper connection that would allow me to explore with Lydia her ambivalence around emotional intimacy and the experience of intense affect.

If I could turn back time, I would be more aware of how my conflictual early relationship with my father led to my readily identifying with Lydia as the victim of a man's aggression and increased my sensitivity to Vincent's rage. At times, my own feelings of anger toward Vincent caused me to respond with an intensity that made Lydia feel defensive of her husband and resulted in her shutting down her own emerging feelings of anger. My sensitivity to Vincent's bullying behavior also caused me to initially see the couple through the black-and-white lens of victim and perpetrator. It took some time for me to understand the extent of Lydia's role in their turbulent relationship and to help her become aware of how she provoked and emotionally injured her husband.

Finally, if I could turn back time, I would be more aware of the healing process that was occurring between Lydia and me, what Karen (2012) refers to as "beckoning." Karen defines beckoning as a process in which "the analyst's growth pulls the patient toward a similar growth" (2012, p. 301). As I unconsciously became more able to integrate my old feelings of hurt and rage with strong feelings of love for my father, I was consciously helping Lydia learn to integrate her feelings of rage and hate toward her husband with her feelings of love for him. Had our work continued, I would have also focused on helping her integrate her dissociated feelings of anger and disappointment toward her father with her idealized image of him.

Awareness of the mutual healing that occurred through my work with Lydia also reflects Aron and Atlas's concept of generative enactments (2015). During the time Lydia and I worked together, she seemed to unconsciously sense my struggle to integrate painful feelings from my childhood as she struggled to give voice to her fury at her husband while still holding onto her love for him. This was an exceptionally trying time for both of us, and though I didn't fully recognize it in our moments together, Lydia and I helped each other hold the messiness and complexity of simply being human and grow from it.

References

Aron, L., & Atlas, G. (2015). Generative enactment: Memories from the future. *Psychoanalytic Dialogues*, 25(3): 309–324.

Gardner, J. (2024). Forms and transformations of empathy: Subtleties and complexities of empathic communication. *Psychoanalysis, Self, and Context*, 19: 80–93.

Gerson, B. (ed.). (1996). *The therapist as a person: Life choices, life experiences, and their effects on treatment*. Routledge.

Karen, R. (2012). Beckoning: The analyst's growth as a therapeutic agent. *Contemporary Psychoanalysis*, 48: 301–328.

Conclusion

I am grateful to the courageous men and women who fill these stories. Our time together has deeply impacted me as a clinician and as a person. They taught me patience, flexibility, understanding, humility, and acceptance. Mandy and Nicki allowed me into their dark and lonely inner worlds and silently permitted me to help them through the worst moments of their young lives. Though I clamored for them to talk about what was distressing and destabilizing them, I eventually learned the value of simply being with another while wordlessly sharing the sharpest edges of their pain. My work with Jamie and Brian showed me the dangerous lure of my own omnipotence and the blinding effect that my longing to heal can sometimes have. Jen and Claire reminded me about the limits of my ability to truly know the inner experience of another and forced me to confront my own difficulty with anger and acceptance. My work with Josh, Daphne, and Evan taught me to be mindful of how my conscious and unconscious experience can silently seep into the world that I share with my patients. Their stories showed me how this infiltration can bring moments of unexpected closeness but can also derail the treatment at its most critical crossroads. And my work with Lydia taught me to acknowledge my own limitations and recognize when I simply don't have one hundred percent to give.

These stories describe how a therapist's full spectrum of emotions, both positive and negative, inevitably influence the treatment process. They highlight the need for us, as clinicians, to understand our own unconscious dynamics, including how our emotional needs and sequestered self-states can unexpectedly take center stage, create blind spots, and affect our clinical work. I still wince when I think about my irritation and impatience with Jen and how this played a role in her abruptly ending treatment. I am struck by waves of grief when I remember Lydia's focus on her husband's rage and his father's rage during those awful months surrounding my father's death. I still beam with pride when I think of Nicki, the warrior child, who will soon be a Ph.D. And then there's Jamie, now four years sober, who I am fortunate to be working with again. Her very presence in the room fills me with hope and reminds me how the fruits of our work can continue to be healing for years to come.

DOI: 10.4324/9781003543343-11

The work we do is not for the faint of heart. We need to be bold enough to tap into the full range of our emotional register and dive into our own psychology so that our passion and our pain are available to us as clinicians. When we bring our whole selves into the treatment room, we become more spontaneous, authentic, and emotionally available to our patients. As we prioritize the misattunements, ruptures, and enactments that inevitably arise between our patients and ourselves, we discover hidden parts of them that are at the center of their stories of pain and conflict but had previously been unreachable. And we gain access to sequestered parts of each of us that we may feel have no business in the treatment room but show up nonetheless.

Now that we are at the end of our road together, I'd like to offer three takeaways from this collection of case studies that are at the heart of my clinical work.

First, our patients need to feel that we care deeply about them and their struggles. While I believe that insightful interpretations are helpful and the experience of feeling understood is crucial, little deep healing will occur unless a patient feels that they truly matter to their therapist.

Second, spontaneity and authenticity lend our clinical understanding the power to move emotional mountains. While they can generate feelings of closeness and trust, they can also result in the misattunements, ruptures, and enactments that can jeopardize the treatment. But by embracing our fallibility, owning our missteps, expressing concern about how we have impacted our patients, and providing more empathic responses, we create new relational experiences for our patients – experiences that are powerful agents of change.

Third, we cannot do deep clinical work from the safety of our analytic perch. We need to meet our patients in the eye of their emotional storm and be willing to feel the intensity of their fear and pain. When we accept that our "therapist selves" won't always be in the driver's seat, we can harness the power of our own inner world to help our patients not only survive their storm but to emerge stronger from it.

Index